Olfa ZOUKAR

# Uterine rupture in 60 cases

Olfa ZOUKAR

# Uterine rupture in 60 cases

## Experience of the Monastir Maternity Centre, Tunisia

ScienciaScripts

**Imprint**

Any brand names and product names mentioned in this book are subject to trademark, brand or patent protection and are trademarks or registered trademarks of their respective holders. The use of brand names, product names, common names, trade names, product descriptions etc. even without a particular marking in this work is in no way to be construed to mean that such names may be regarded as unrestricted in respect of trademark and brand protection legislation and could thus be used by anyone.

Cover image: www.ingimage.com

This book is a translation from the original published under ISBN 978-620-3-45334-8.

Publisher:
Sciencia Scripts
is a trademark of
Dodo Books Indian Ocean Ltd. and OmniScriptum S.R.L publishing group

120 High Road, East Finchley, London, N2 9ED, United Kingdom
Str. Armeneasca 28/1, office 1, Chisinau MD-2012, Republic of Moldova, Europe
Printed at: see last page
**ISBN: 978-620-7-30105-8**

# Contents

# 1 Introduction

Uterine rupture is an obstetric emergency defined as a non-surgical rupture of the uterine wall during pregnancy or labour [1].

A distinction should be made between complete uterine rupture, which is characterised by damage to the entire uterine wall (endometrium, myometrium and serosa), and incomplete or partial rupture, which is defined as dehiscence of the endometrium and myometrium without damage to the uterine serosa.

Although uterine rupture has become exceptional in developed countries, with a prevalence of 0.5/10,000 to 7.9/10,000 births [2], it remains the prerogative of under-medicalised countries. Its frequency depends on the quality of pregnancy monitoring and delivery management, and therefore on the human and material resources and infrastructure available.

Inflation in cesarean section rates over the last 20 years and the use of uterine testing have contributed to an increase in the risk of uterine rupture [3]. Other risk factors are thought to be involved, such as induction of labour, use of prostaglandins, advanced maternal age, prolonged term of pregnancy, presence of a myomectomy scar and short intergenital interval [3].

Uterine rupture in a healthy uterus is a much less frequent event. Its prevalence is estimated at between 1/17,000 and 1/20,000 deliveries, and its maternal and fatal prognosis is poorer [4].

Uterine rupture is a dreadful obstetric complication, with a high maternal and fatal mortality rate, especially in the case of a healthy uterus, due to a possible delay in diagnosis and inadequate management [5]. It is a typical medical, surgical and obstetric emergency. Its prognosis depends closely on the speed and quality of management. The frequency of uterine rupture is therefore a good indicator of the degree of medicalisation in a country.

In our country, uterine rupture remains a relatively frequent complication, making a major contribution to maternal mortality through the associated haemorrhage. Haemorrhage remains the leading cause of maternal death, despite prevention efforts, in particular through the national perinatal programme (PNP) [6].

Directives have been issued to first-degree maternity hospitals limiting the level of care and, a fortiori, the frequency of obstetric complications. However, this attitude has resulted in an increased workload for university maternity hospitals and inadequate human and material resources.

In addition, the rate of cesarean section is constantly increasing, reaching 26.7% in 2011 [7], which raises questions about the associated risk of uterine rupture. All this justifies our interest in this pathology.

We have therefore set ourselves the following objectives:

-To determine the epidemiological profile of patients with uterine rupture.

-To describe the management methods and maternal and fatal prognosis for uterine rupture.

## 1. Type and location of study

This is a cross-sectional, descriptive and analytical, single-centre retrospective study conducted in the obstetric gynecology department of the Monastir maternity and neonatology centre (CMNM) over a 5-year period from 01/01/2017 to 31/12/2021.

## 2. Study population

### 2.1. Inclusion criteria

All cases of uterine rupture (complete or incomplete) in healthy and scarred uteri in pregnant women of any term in the obstetric gynaecology department of the CMNM during the study period.

### 2.2. Non-inclusion criteria

- All cases of considerable thinning of a uterine scar during an operative cesarean section or uterine revision after vaginal delivery

- Tears limited to the uterine cervix, uterine perforations during abortion and placenta accreta.

### 2.3. Exclusion criteria

- Patients with incomplete or unusable records.

## 3. Data collection

Data was collected retrospectively from the patients' medical records and operative report books. For each patient, we drew up a data collection form (**Appendix 1**) designed for the purposes of this study.

This sheet contains the following items:

### 3.1. Clinical data

The main clinical data are

- **Epidemiological data** (age, origin, civil status, medical and surgical antecedents).

- **Obstetrical history** (pregnancy, parity, abortion, voluntary termination of pregnancy (IVP), number of cesarean sections, indications and terms of any previous cesarean sections).

- **Gynecological history** (endo uterine procedures: aspiration-curettage, uterine revision).

- **Pregnancy-related data** (pregnancy follow-up, number of ANCs, screening for GDM, quality of obstetric pelvis, ultrasound data from the $1^{ier}$ , 2 '-th and $3^{i\text{-me}}$ trimesters)

- **Clinical examination** (circumstances of discovery, gestational age, intergenital interval, time of discovery, bishop score, progress of labour, lesion investigations: type and age of RU, mode of delivery).

### 3.2. Therapeutic methods used

- Resuscitation elements (hemodynamic status, transfusion with number of packed red blood cells and units of fresh frozen plasma, biological results)
- Conservative treatment
- Radical treatment (total or subtotal hysterectomy).
- Therapeutic abstention

### 3.3. Prognostic elements

- Maternal prognosis (maternal mortality, intraoperative complications, postoperative complications)
- Fatal prognosis (fatal weight and APGAR score at birth, transfer to neonatology department, early neonatal death)

To assess the medium-term prognosis, the patients included were contacted by telephone at least 6 months after delivery. The response rate was 80%. A questionnaire was drawn up containing 12 questions (**Appendix 2**).

### 4. Statistical analysis

All data entry and statistical analysis were carried out using Microsoft Office Excel 2019 and IBMSPSS.

### 4.1. Descriptive study

We calculated the numbers and frequencies (percentages) used to describe the categorical variables.

For quantitative variables, the distribution of the data was studied using skewness and kurtosis coefficients and tests of normality. These variables were described by means and standard deviation in the case of a normal distribution and by medians and quartiles in the opposite case.

### 4.2. Analytical study

To analyse the association between two qualitative variables, we used Pearson's $\chi^2$ test to compare two frequencies if the conditions of application were verified, and Fischer's test if they were not.

For the analysis of the association between two quantitative variables, we used the *STUDENT* test for the comparison of two means and the *ANOVA* test for the comparison of several means in the case of a normal distribution, and respectively the non-parametric *MANN WITNEY* and Kruskal Wallis tests in the opposite case. We used the significance level for $p < 5\%$.

### 5. Bibliographical research

The bibliographic search was carried out by consulting computerised bibliographic databases (pubmed, cochrane library, google scholar, science direct) and postgraduate courses using the following key words: uterine rupture, scarred uterus, non-scarred uterus, dehiscence, prognosis.

## 6. Ethical considerations and conflicts of interest

This study was carried out in compliance with ethical standards in research, i.e. anonymity and confidentiality of data, and presents no conflict of interest.

# 3 Results

## 1. Descriptive study

### 1.1. Flow chart :

During the study period (2017-2021) we recorded 61 cases of uterine rupture out of a total of 28546 deliveries, i.e. a rate of 2.13 ^ **(Figure 1).**

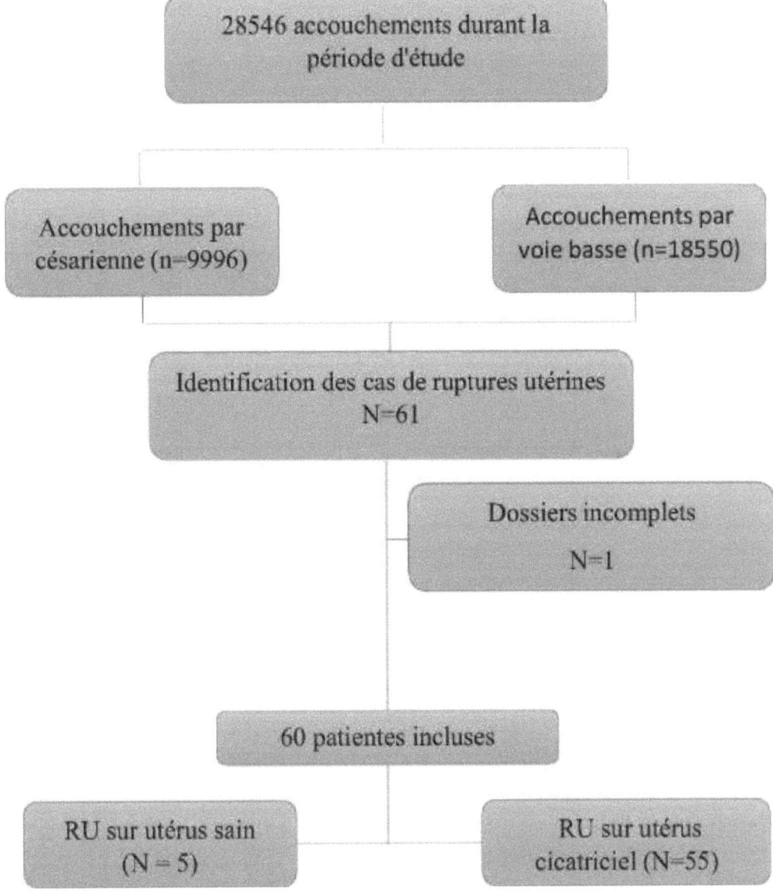


**Figure 1: Patient selection flow chart**

### 1.2. Prevalence of uterine rupture by year of study :

The caesarean section rate was 35.1%, i.e. one for every 2.85 deliveries. During this period, there was an increase in the rate of ruptures from 1.**43%** to 4.65%, as well as an increase in the rate of cesarean deliveries from 32% to 42.4% (**Table I**).

**Table I: Prevalence of mode of delivery and uterine rupture between 2017 and 2021.**

| Year | Number of births | Delivery by vaginal route | | Delivery by cesarean section | | Uterine rupture | |
|---|---|---|---|---|---|---|---|
| | | N | % | N | % | N | % |
| 2017 | 6284 | 4278 | 68.0 | 2006 | 32.0 | 9 | *1.43* |
| 2018 | 6206 | 4202 | 67.7 | 2004 | 32.3 | 10 | 1.61 |
| 2019 | 6273 | 4091 | 65.2 | 2182 | 34.8 | 9 | 1.43 |
| 2020 | 5257 | 3372 | 64.1 | 1885 | 35.9 | 11 | 2.09 |
| 2021 | 4526 | 2607 | 57.6 | 1919 | 42.4 | 21 | 4.65 |
| Total | 28546 | 18550 | 64.9 | 9996 | 35.1 | 60 | 2.10 |

Of the 60 cases of UR, 55 occurred in a scar uterus, with a maximum frequency of 21 cases recorded in 2021 (**Figure 2**).

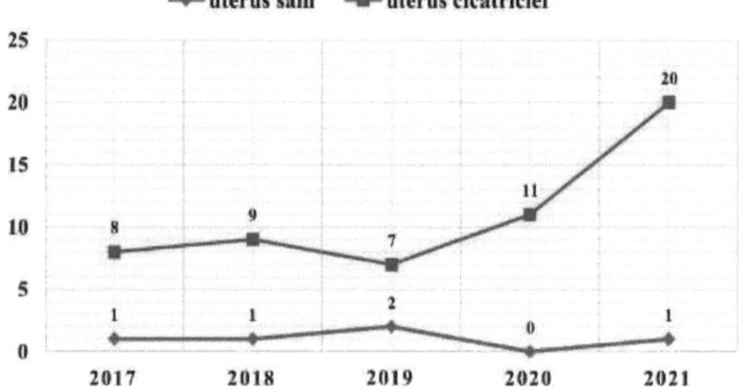

Year

**Figure 2: Distribution of uterine ruptures by year of study.**

### 1.3. Epidemiological profile of patients

### 1.3.1. Age of patients

The average maternal age was 30.88±0.635, with extremes of 18 and 42 years. The age group most affected was between 26 and 30 years. Uterine rupture occurred in patients aged over 30 in 52.7% of cases, with 3 cases in healthy uteruses and 28 in scar uteruses (**Table II**).

**Table II: Distribution of uterine ruptures according to patient age.**

| Maternal age | RU on healthy uterus | | RU on scar uterus | | Total | |
|---|---|---|---|---|---|---|
| | N | % | N | % | N | % |
| < 20 | 0 | 0,0 | 1 | 1,8 | 1 | 1,7 |
| 21-25 | 2 | 40,0 | 7 | 12,6 | 9 | 15,3 |
| 26-30 | 0 | 0,0 | 19 | 34,2 | 19 | 32,3 |
| 31-35 | 2 | 40,0 | 15 | 27,0 | 17 | 28,9 |
| 36-40 | 1 | 20,0 | 11 | 19,8 | 12 | 20,4 |
| > 41 | 0 | 0,0 | 2 | 3,6 | 2 | 3,4 |

| Mean ±ESM | 30,80 ± 2,083 | 30,89 ± 0,672 | 30,88 ±0,635 |

### 1.3.2. Pregnancy follow-up

For the healthy uterus group (n=5), two patients, or 40%, were correctly monitored (number of antenatal visits greater than or equal to 4), compared with three patients, or 60%, who were poorly monitored.

In the scar uterus group, 38 patients (69.1%) were well monitored, compared with 17 patients (30.9%) who were poorly monitored (Table III).

**Table III: Distribution of RU according to the number of antenatal consultations.**

| Number of consultations | RU on healthy uterus N | % | RU on scar uterus N | % | Total N | % |
|---|---|---|---|---|---|---|
| 0 | 0 | 0,0 | 0 | 0,0 | 0 | 0,0 |
| 1a 3 | 3 | 60,0 | 17 | 30,9 | 19 | 31,66 |
| >4 | 2 | 40,0 | 38 | 69,1 | 41 | 68,33 |

### 1.3.3. Origins of patients

The patients in our study were divided into 36 women of urban origin (60% of cases) and 24 of rural origin (40% of cases).

### 1.4. Patient history

### 1.4.1. Medical history

A medical history of gestational diabetes was present in 5 patients, or 8% of cases. In addition, four patients (6.6%) had a history of hypertension (Table IV).

**Table IV: Patients' medical history.**

| Medical history | RU on healthy uterus N | % | N | RU on scar uterus % | Total N | % |
|---|---|---|---|---|---|---|
| Diabetes | 0 | 0,0 | 5 | 9,0 | 5 | 8,3 |
| HTA | 1 | 20,0 | 3 | 5,5 | 4 | 6,6 |
| Other | 0 | 0,0 | 4 | 7,2 | 4 | 6,6 |

### 1.4.2. Previous surgery

Seven patients had a surgical antecedent of myomectomy, a rate of 11.6%. One patient had a history of hysteroplasty and one had a history of salpingectomy (Table V).

**Table V: Breakdown of patients' surgical antecedents.**

| Surgical history | RU on healthy uterus N | % | RU on scar uterus N | % | Total N | % |
|---|---|---|---|---|---|---|
| Myomectomy | 0 | 0,0 | 7 | 12,7 | 7 | 11,6 |
| Hysteroplasty | 0 | 0,0 | 1 | 1,8 | 1 | 1,6 |
| Salpingectomy | 0 | 0,0 | 1 | 1,8 | 1 | 1,6 |
| Other | 1 | 20,0 | 3 | 5,5 | 4 | 6,7 |

### 1.4.3. Gynecological history

The antecedent uterine revision was found in three cases and aspiration for voluntary termination of pregnancy in ten cases **(Table VI).**

**Table VI: Breakdown of patients' gynaecological antecedents.**

| Gynaecological history | RU on healthy uterus | | RU on scar uterus | | Total | |
|---|---|---|---|---|---|---|
| | N | % | N | % | N | % |
| Uterine revision | 1 | 20,0 | 2 | 3,6 | 3 | 5,0 |
| Suction for abortion | 1 | 20,0 | 9 | 16,3 | 10 | 16,6 |
| Other | 0 | 0,0 | 4 | 7,2 | 4 | 6,6 |

### 1.4.4. Obstetrical history

#### 1.4.4.1. Parite maternelle

The mean parity for the study population was 2.57 divided into 3.6 for patients in the healthy uterus group and 2.47 for those in the scar uterus group **(Table VII).**

**Table VII: Breakdown of uterine ruptures by patient category**

| Parite | RU on healthy uterus | | RU on scar uterus | | Total | |
|---|---|---|---|---|---|---|
| | N | % | N | % | N | % |
| 1 | 0 | 0 | 0 | 0,0 | 0 | 0,0 |
| 2 | 1 | 20 | 33 | 60,0 | 34 | 56,7 |
| 3 | 1 | 20 | 19 | 34,5 | 21 | 35,0 |
| 4 | 2 | 40 | 2 | 3,7 | 3 | 5,0 |
| 5 | 1 | 20 | 1 | 1,8 | 2 | 3,3 |
| Mean ±ESM | 3,6 ± 0,51 | | 2,47 ± 0,09 | | 2,57 ± 0,1 | |
| Mediane | 4 | | 2 | | 2 | |

The majority of cases of rupture in a scarred uterus have involved paraplegics. Of the cases of UR in a healthy uterus, 60% were multiparous **(Figure 3).**

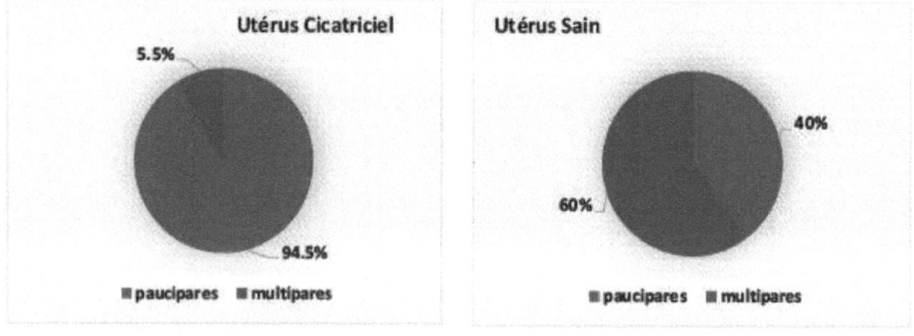


**Figure 3: Distribution of patients according to uterine condition**

#### 1.4.4.2. History of caesarean section:

The average total number of previous caesarean sections was 1.51
Forty-five patients had uni- scar uteri, a percentage of 75%, and 10 patients had bi- or multi-scar uteri, a percentage of 16.7% **(Figure 4)**.

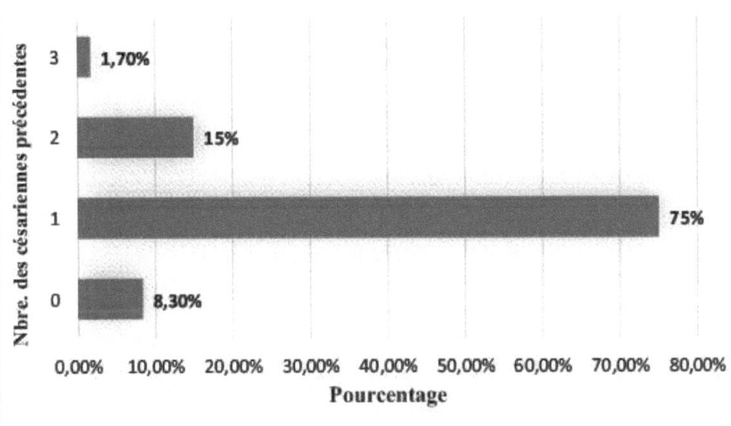


**Figure 4: Distribution of patients according to previous caesarean section** 1.4.4.3
**Intergenital interval**

The mean intergenital interval for patients with scar uteri was 13.4 months, with extremes ranging from 4 months to 5 years. Four patients (7.2%) had an intergenital interval of less than or equal to 6 months **(Figure 5)**.

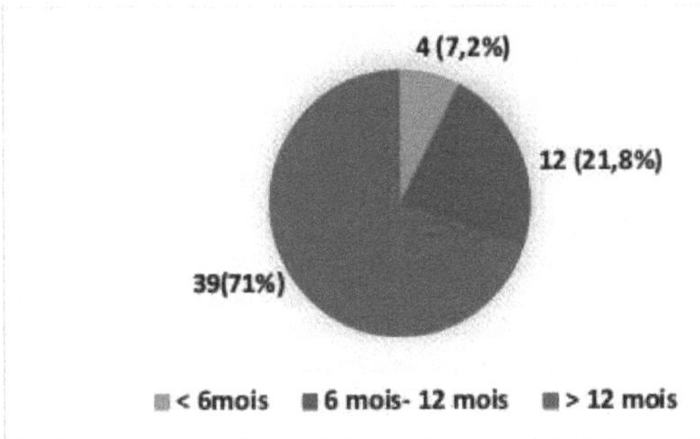


**Figure 5: Distribution of patients according to intergenital interval.**

1.4.4.4 **Indication of previous cesarean section**

The most common indications for previous cesarean section were stagnation of dilatation in 18.3% of cases and SFA in 16.7% **(Figure 6)**.

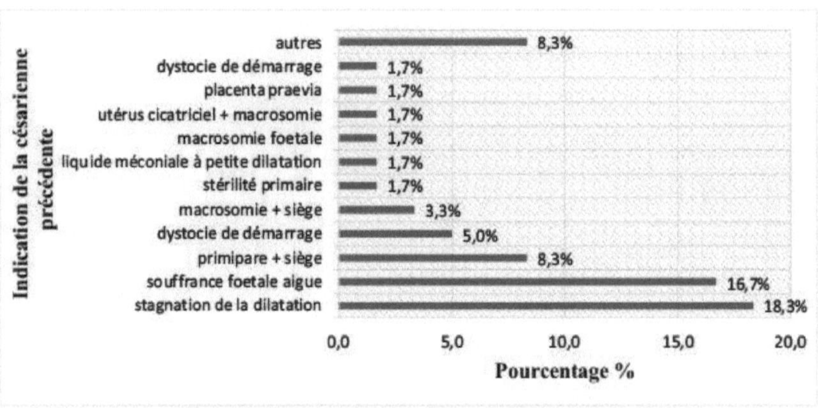


**Figure 6. Distribution of patients according to indication for previous cesarean section.**

## 1.5. Clinical and radiological characteristics :

### 1.5.1. Patient BMI

For the 60 cases of UR, 20% of patients were of normal build (BMI between 18 and 25) compared with 38.3% overweight (BMI between 25 and 30) and 41.6% obese (BMI > 30) **(Table VIII)**.

**Table VIII: Breakdown of uterine ruptures according to the MCL of the patients.**

| Patient BMI | RU on healthy uterus | | RU on scar uterus | | Total | |
|---|---|---|---|---|---|---|
| | N | % | N | % | N | % |
| 18-25 | 0 | 0,0 | 12 | 21,8 | 12 | 20,0 |
| 25-30 | 1 | 20,0 | 22 | 40,0 | 23 | 38,3 |
| 30-35 | 3 | 60,0 | 20 | 36,4 | 23 | 38,3 |
| > 35 | 1 | 20,0 | 1 | 1,8 | | 23,3 |
| Mean ±ESM | 34,55 ± 3,03 | | 28,43 ± 0,57 | | 28,94 ± 0,61 | |
| Mediane | 33,8 | | 29,4 | | 29,4 | |

### 1.5.2. Examination of the pelvis

Nine patients had a pathological pelvis, divided into 8 patients with scarred uteri, i.e. a rate of 14.54%, and one with a healthy uterus, i.e. 20%.

### 1.5.3. Ultrasound data

We noted 7 dystocic presentations, divided into 2 transverse presentations and 5 seat presentations. Pregnancies were monofetal in 96% of cases with 2 gemellar bi-chorionic bi-amniotic pregnancies **(Table IX)**.

**Table IX: Obstetric ultrasound data**

| Ultrasound data | | RU on healthy uterus | | RU on scar uterus | |
|---|---|---|---|---|---|
| | | N | % | N | % |
| | Cephalic | 5 | 100 | 50 | 87,7 |
| Presentation | Transverse | 0 | 0,0 | 2 | 3,5 |

| | | N | % | N | % |
|---|---|---|---|---|---|
| **Quantity of liquid** | Seat | 0 | 0,0 | 5 | 8,7 |
| | Oligohydramnios | 1 | 20,0 | 14 | 24,56 |
| | Hydramnios | 0 | 0,0 | 2 | 3,5 |
| | Normal | 4 | 80,0 | 41 | 71,92 |
| **Type of pregnancy** | Monofetal | 100 | 100 | 53 | 96,4 |
| | Multiple | 0 | 0.0 | 2 | 3,6 |

## 1.6. Moment of rupture and circumstances of discovery

RU was discovered before term in 5 patients and at a term *>37* SA in 55 patients, i.e. frequencies of 8.3% and 91.7% respectively **(Table X)**.

**Table X: Breakdown of uterine ruptures by term of pregnancy**

| Term of pregnancy (SA) | RU on healthy uterus | | RU on scar uterus | | Total |
|---|---|---|---|---|---|
| | N | % | N | % | N% |
| From 27 to 37 | 0 | 0,0 | 5 | 9,1 | 58,3 |
| From 37 to 41 | 3 | 60,0 | 37 | 67,3 | 4066,7 |
| From 41 to 42 | 1 | 20,0 | 13 | 23,6 | 1423,3 |
| > 42 | 1 | 20,0 | 0 | 0,0 | 11,7 |

### 1.6.1. Pre-term uterine rupture (before 37 weeks' gestation) :

There were five cases of preterm RU in scar uteri, i.e. 8.3%. One case involved a bi-scar uterus and four cases involved patients with a uni-scar uterus. Gestational age ranged from 34 to 36 weeks' gestation. The pregnancy was poorly monitored in only one patient.

One of the patients had a history of gestational diabetes **(Table XI)**.

**Table XI: Characteristics of cases of uterine rupture occurring before term**

| Case No. / Features | 1 | 2 | 3 | 4 | 5 |
|---|---|---|---|---|---|
| Age | 38 | 42 | 29 | 38 | 27 |
| Parite | 2 | 3 | 2 | 2 | 2 |
| Number of scars | 1 | 2 | 1 | 1 | 1 |
| BMI | 29,5 | 33,1 | 26 | 33 | 29,2 |
| Gestational age (SA) | 34 | 36 | 34+5days | 35 | 36 |
| Clinical symptoms | SFA | Metrorragie | SFA | SFA | SFA |
| A moment of discovery | Before work | Before work | Phase of latency | Before work | Phase of latency |
| Fatal Weight | 2100 | 3400 | 1780 | 4500 | 3300 |
| Apgar score | 5/5/6 | 9/1/10 | 7/7/8 | Deaths | 5/8/9 |
| RU headquarters | Segment Lower | Segment Lower | Segmento body | Segmento-body | Segmento-body |
| Treatment | Suture | Suture | Suture | Hysterectomy | Suture |

The clinical signs found were: pathological RCF in four patients and metrorrhagia related to placenta previa in another. All patients delivered by cesarean section. The uterine rupture was segmental-corporeal and complete in 3 cases and incomplete segmental in 2 cases. The birth weights of the newborns ranged from 1700 g to 3400 g. There was only one case of macrosomia in a stillborn weighing 4500g. Treatment was conservative surgery in 4 patients.

A case of hysterectomy in the face of postpartum haemorrhage resistant to medical treatment was recorded in a second parous patient undergoing caesarean section for a pathological RCF at 35 weeks' gestation **(Table XII)**.

### 1.6.2. Ruptured uterus at term (> 37 SA)

**1.6.2.1. Breakdown by term of pregnancy at time of discovery**

Forty cases of UR occurred at term between 37 and 41 days' gestation, i.e. 66.7%, three of which occurred in a healthy uterus. RU was prolonged in 14 patients, one of whom had a healthy uterus and the others had scar uteri **(Table XI)**.

**1.6.2.2. Clinical symptoms**

We noted an abnormal FHR in 27 patients, i.e. a rate of 49.1%, and metrorrhagia during labour in 9, i.e. a frequency of 16.3%. Six patients were asymptomatic **(Table XII)**.

Table XII: Clinical circumstances in which UR is discovered at term.

| Clinical signs | RU on healthy uterus | | RU on scar uterus | | Total | |
|---|---|---|---|---|---|---|
| | N | % | N | % | N | % |
| RCF abnormality | 2 | 40,0 | 25 | 50,0 | 27 | 49,1 |
| Abdominal pain | 0 | 0,0 | 3 | 6,0 | | 35,5 |
| Metrorrhagia during labour | 1 | 20,0 | 8 | 16,0 | 9 | 16,3 |
| Uterine hypercinesia | 0 | 0,0 | 5 | 10,0 | | 59,1 |
| | 1 | 20,0 | 2 | 4,0 | 3 | 5,5 |
| Postpartum metrorrhagia | 1 | 20,0 | 1 | 2,0 | 2 | 3,6 |
| Asymptomatic | 0 | 0,0 | 6 | 12,0 | 6 | 10,9 |

**1.6.2.3. Time to discover the UK**

***Outside labour****:* Seven cases of RU out of 55 occurred before the onset of labour, i.e. a rate of 12.7%. We discovered three cases of rupture in patients with a single scar uterus during an emergency cesarean section in the presence of a pathological RCF, and four cases during a cesarean section planned for a bi-scar uterus **(Table XIII)**.

***During labour****:* We recorded 43 cases of RU during labour: 53% of cases occurred during the latency phase, 37% were discovered during the active phase and only 4 cases were completely dilated. Patients with a single scar uterus accounted for 74.5% of cases of uterine rupture at term, 80% of which were discovered during the latency and active phases **(Table XIIITable XIII).**

**Table XIII: Time of discovery of forward URs**

| A moment of discovery | Number of scars before RU | | | | Total | |
| --- | --- | --- | --- | --- | --- | --- |
| | **0** | **1** | **2** | **3** | **N** | **%** |
| **Before work** | 0 | 3 | 4 | 0 | 7 | 12,7 |
| **Latency phase** | 1 | 18 | 3 | 1 | 23 | 41,8 |
| **Active phase** | 0 | 15 | 1 | 0 | 16 | 29 |
| **Complete expansion** | 2 | 2 | 0 | 0 | | 47,2 |
| **Systematic post uterine revision** | 0 | 2 | 0 | 0 | | 23,6 |
| **Partum Delivery haemorrhage** | 1 | 1 | 0 | 0 | | 23,6 |
| **Unstable hemodynamic state** | 1 | 0 | 0 | 0 | | 11,8 |

***Immediate postpartum***: In the postpartum period we recorded 5 cases of rupture, a rate of 8.3%. For patients with a single scar uterus, uterine rupture was discovered during a systematic uterine revision for two patients and following the appearance of a delivery hemorrhage for one patient.

other. For patients with a healthy uterus, uterine rupture was diagnosed after delivery in 2 cases: one case died following the onset of delivery haemorrhage and the other in the presence of the onset of haemorrhagic shock.

1.6.2.4. **Characteristics of labour and delivery in cases of full-term RU**

In the scar uterus group, labour was induced in 22% of cases compared with 80% in the healthy uterus group. The mean durations of the active phase for the healthy uterus and scar uterus groups were 0.57 and 2.86 hours respectively **(Table XIV).**

**Table XIV: Characteristics of labour and mode of delivery in cases of uterine rupture at term**

| Features | RU on healthy uterus N | RU on scar uterus N |
| --- | --- | --- |
| **Spontaneous work** | 1 | 39 |
| **Induced Labour** | 4 | 11 |
| *DPIO* | 1 | 6 |
| **Mode of** *Misoprostol* | 2 | 0 |
| *Dinoprostone* | 1 | 0 |
| *SEA* **trip** | 0 | 5 |
| **Mode** *Normal AVB* | 2 | 3 |
| *Forceps* **delivery** | 0 | 2 |
| *Emergency CS* | 3 | 45 |
| **Oxytocin infusion** | 3 | 0 |
| *< 3000* | 0 | 14 |
| **Deadly weight** *3000-4000* | 2 | 30 |
| *>4000* | 3 | 8 |
| ***Fatal weight Mean (grams)*** | 4000 *grams* | 3200 *grams* |

| Average duration of the latency phase | 10.4 hours | 7.9 hours |
| Average length of active phase | 0.57 hours | 2.8 hours |
| Duration of the opening of the auf | 5.16 hours | 6 hours |

Of the 5 patients with a healthy uterus, two underwent normal vaginal delivery and 3 underwent emergency cesarean delivery in response to an abnormal FFR. In the group of women with a scarred uterus, 45 delivered by emergency cesarean section and 2 delivered by forceps in the presence of fetal bradycardia. The different indications for emergency cesarean section are detailed in the following figure **(Figure 7).**

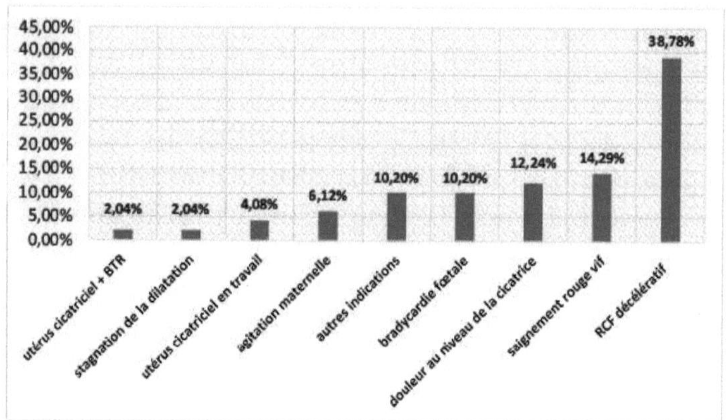


Figure 7. Frequency of indications for emergency cesarean section

### 1.6.2.5. Uterine rupture in a healthy uterus :

The average maternal age was 30.8, with extremes of 24 and 40 years. Sixty per cent of the women were multiparous.

All cases of RU in a healthy uterus occurred at term and during labour. Two cases were discovered in the post-partum period: one following the onset of maternal hypotension and the other following the onset of metrorrhagia.

Labour was induced in 80% of cases, and the most common clinical sign was an abnormal FHR. The rupture was segmental-corporeal in 2 cases and corporeal in 3 cases. Hysterectomy was performed in 2 patients, i.e. in 40% of cases **(Table XV).**

**Table XV: Characteristics of uterine rupture in healthy uterus**

| Case No. | 1 | 2 | 3 | 4 | 5 |
|---|---|---|---|---|---|
| Age | 24 | 32 | 25 | 33 | 40 |
| Parite | 2 | 3 | 4 | 4 | 5 |
| BMI | 34,9 | 31,1 | 27,6 | 45,7 | 33,2 |
| Gestational age | 39 | 40 | 42SA+1dr | 41SA+3dr | 40SA+1dr |

16

| Clinical signs | Metrorragie | EHD Unstable | Metrorragie | Anomaly of RCF | RCF abnormality |
|---|---|---|---|---|---|
| Moment of discovery | Phase of Latency | Post Partum | Post partum | Expansion complete | Expansion complete |
| Work release | Dinoprostone | Nothing | Misoprostol | DPIO | Misoprostol |
| Deadly weight | 3900 | 3500 | 4000 | 4400 | 4200 |
| Apgar | 6/6/9 | 7/7/8 Transfer | 6/6/8 | Decede | Decede |
| Type of break | Incomplete | Complete | Complete | Complete | Complete |
| Treatment | Suture | Hysterectomy | Suture | Hysterectomy | Suture + LT |

## 1.7. Anatomical lesions

### 1.7.1. Anatomical type of lesion

UC was incomplete in 37 cases, i.e. a frequency of 61.7%, and complete in 23 cases, i.e. in 38.3% of cases of rupture. Twenty per cent of ruptures in healthy uteruses were incomplete, compared with 65.5% in scar uteruses.

### 1.7.2. Location of lesions

The uterine rupture was segmental in 43 cases, i.e. 71.6% of the total number of ruptures, segmentocorporeal in 14 cases, i.e. 23.3%, and corporeal in 3 cases, i.e. 5% of cases **(Figure 8)**. In cases involving a scar uterus, the rupture was segmental in 43 cases and segmentocorporeal in 12 cases.

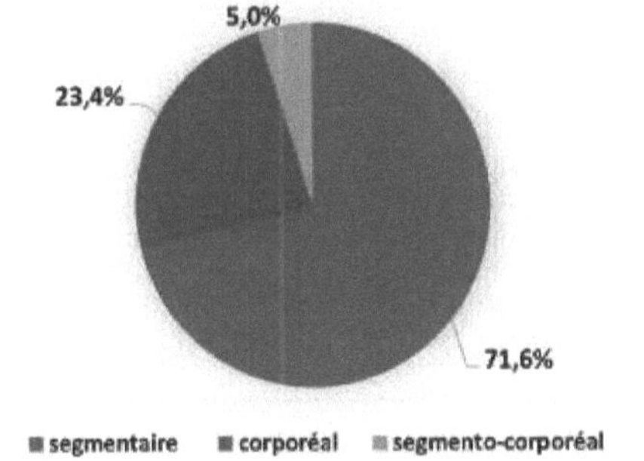


**Figure 8. Breakdown of RUs by location of rupture.**

### 1.7.3. Associated lesions

The associated lesions were mainly a bladder sore in 10% of cases and a cervical tear in 8.3% **(Figure 9)**.

Six patients presented with bladder lesions, five of whom had scar uteri.

All vaginal lesions occurred in patients with healthy uteri. Cervical lesions occurred in two patients with scar uteri following instrumental delivery and in 3 patients with healthy uteri.

d'utérus sain.

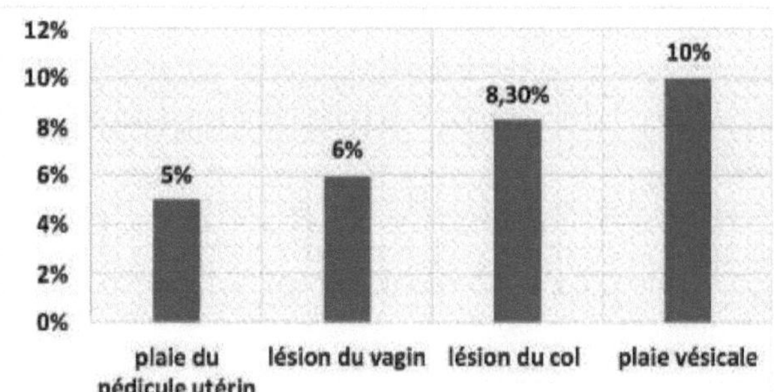


**Figure 9. Lesions associated with uterine rupture**

**Table XVI** summarises the anamnestic, clinical and operative features of the UR cases in our study.

**Table XVI. Epidemiological and clinical characteristics of the patients in our study**

| Features | Healthy uterus N=5 | Scarred uteri N=55 |
|---|---|---|
| Average age of patients | 30,80 ± 2,083 | 30,89 ± 0,672 |
| Average gestational age | 40,3±0.62 | 39.19+0.22 |
| Gestational age > 41 SA | 2(40%) | 13(23,6%) |
| Medium parity | 3.6+0.51 | 2.47+0.089 |
| Average BMI | 34,55 ± 3,03 | 28,43 ± 0,57 |
| Number of previous cesarean sections | | |
| 0 | 5 | 0 |
| 1 | 0 | 45(82%) |
| >1 | 0 | 10(18%) |
| History of myomectomy | 0 | 7(12.72%) |
| Multiple pregnancy | 0 | 2(3.36%) |
| Boundary basin | 1(20%) | 8(14.54%) |
| Dystocic presentation | 0 | 7(12.8%) |
| Hydramnios | 0 | 2(3.6%) |
| Macrosomia (fetal weight > 4KG) | 3(60%) | 9(16%) |
| Clinical signs | | |
| RCF abnormality | 2(40%) | 29(52,7%) |
| Metrorragie | 2(40%) | 10(18%) |
| A moment of discovery | | |
| Outside work | 0 | 10(18.2%) |
| During work | 3(60%) | 42(76.3%) |
| Post partum | 2(40%) | 3(5,5%) |

| | | | |
|---|---|---|---|
| Type of break | | | |
| Complete | | 4(80%) | 19(34,5%) |
| Incomplete | | 1(20%) | 36(65,5%) |
| RU headquarters | | | |
| Segment | | 0 | 43(78,2%) |
| Corporeal | | 100% | 12(21,8%) |

## 1.8. Treatment

### 1.8.1. Resuscitation

Blood transfusions were given to 14 patients. They received an average of 3 packed red blood cells, with extremes ranging from 2 to 6 packed red blood cells. Among patients with a healthy uterus, 60% required resuscitation by blood transfusion, compared with 20% of parturients with a scarred uterus. Four patients received units of fresh frozen plasma in response to a hemostasis disorder, with an average number of 8 and extremes ranging from 4 to 12 units.

### 1.8.2. Surgical treatment

#### 1.8.2.1. Conservative treatment

Conservative treatment was carried out in 56 patients, 53 of whom had a scar uterus **(Table XII)**.

Among the cases of UR treated by suture, tubal sterilisation by tubal ligation was carried out in 9 patients, representing 16% of conservative treatment.

**Table XVII: Distribution of surgical techniques according to the existence of a uterine scar**

| Surgical techniques | RU on healthy uterus | | RU on scar uterus | | Total | |
|---|---|---|---|---|---|---|
| | N | % | N | % | N | % |
| Simple suture | 2 | 40,0 | 45 | 81,8 | 47 | 78,3 |
| Suture + LT | 1 | 20,0 | 8 | 14,5 | 9 | 15,0 |
| Total hysterectomy | 2 | 40,0 | 0 | 0,0 | 2 | 3,3 |
| Subtotal hysterectomy | 0 | 0,0 | 2 | 3,6 | 2 | 3,3 |

#### 1.8.2.2. Radical treatment (hysterectomy):

A hysterectomy for hemostasis was performed in 4 cases (6.6%). Among the 5 cases of RU in a healthy uterus, hemostasis hysterectomy was indicated in 2 cases, i.e. a percentage of 40%. In the case of RU in a scar uterus, hysterectomy for hemostasis was indicated in 2 cases out of 55 **(Table XVIII)**.

**Table XVIII: Profile and clinical context of cases of hysterectomy for hemostasis**

| Name | Age | Parite | Number of scars | Clinical context |
|---|---|---|---|---|
| M.R | 38 | 2 | 1 | Delivery haemorrhage + EDC |
| S.G | 34 | 3 | 2 | Uterine atony |
| R.B | 32 | 3 | 0 | EDC + extended neck wound |
| B.A | 33 | 4 | 0 | EDC + extended neck wound |

# 1.9. Prognosis

## 1.9.1. Maternal prognosis

### 1.9.1.1. Maternal morbidity

***Intraoperative complications:*** We noted 11 cases of RU complicated by haemorrhage. Of these, five patients benefited from triple vascular ligation and one from padding to control the bleeding. In addition, we recorded six cases of intraoperative bladder injury, accounting for 10% of UR.

Four patients developed hemostasis disorders. The mean results of the biological tests were :

- An average prothrombin rate (PT) of 45%,
- An average fibrinemia of 2.6 g/l,
- An average platelet count of 120,000.

***Postoperative complications:*** We recorded anemia in 31.7%, urinary tract infection in 6.7% and functional ileus in 11.7% of the total number of ruptures **(Table XIX)**.

### 1.9.1.2. Maternal mortality

During the study period, no maternal deaths were recorded, giving a mortality rate of 0%.

**Table XIX: Postoperative maternal complications**

| Maternal complications | N | % |
|---|---|---|
| Anemie | 19 | 31,7 |
| Urinary tract infection | 4 | 6,7 |
| Bronchopulmonary infection | 3 | 5,0 |
| Ileus functional | 7 | 11,7 |
| Wound infection | 2 | 3,3 |
| Hospital stay > 5 days | 18 | 30,0 |

## 1.9.2. Perinatal prognosis

### 1.9.2.1. Perinatal morbidity

**Apgar score:** An Apgar score of less than 7 was recorded in 80% of newborns in the healthy uterus rupture group and in 24.5% of newborns in the scar uterus group **(Table XX).**

**Table XX: Breakdown of births by Apgar score**

| Apgar score at 5 min | Number of births to healthy uteruses (n=5) | Number of births with scar uterus (n=57)* |
|---|---|---|
| < 3 | 2(40%) | 1(1.7%) |
| 4a 6 | 2(40%) | 13(22.8%) |
| >7 | 1(20%) | 43(75.5%) |

[*]: the number of births in the case of a scar uterus equals 55 births with two gemellar pregnancies.

<u>**Transfer to the neonatology department:**</u> Of the 7 cases of transfer to the neonatology department, 3 newborns died despite resuscitation, mainly because of neonatal respiratory distress **(Table XXI).**

**Table XXI: Description of cases of newborn babies transferred to the neonatology department**

| Case no. | Uterus | Term (SA) | Pathology during Y | SFA | Apgar 5min | Deadly weight | Morbidity <7j | Mortality <7j |
|---|---|---|---|---|---|---|---|---|
| 1 | Cicatricial | 38 | DG | - | 6 | 4300 | DRNN | - |
| 2j1 | Cicatricial | 37+4j | - | + | 4 | 1700 | DRNN convulsion | Decede |
| 3j2 | Cicatricial | 37+4j | - | + | 7 | 2400 | DRNN | - |
| 4 | Cicatricial | 41+3j | - | + | 4 | 4500 | DRNN APN | Decede |
| 5 | Cicatricial | 40 | DG | + | 6 | 3500 | Suspicion of MFI | - |
| 6 | Healthy | 40 | - | - | 7 | 3500 | Suspicion of MFI | - |
| 7 | Cicatricial | 34 | - | + | 6 | 2100 | DRNN APN | Decede |

**1.9.2.2 : Freight mortality**

In our series, we noted 7 cases of foetal loss, 4 of which occurred per partum and 3 after transfer to the neonatology department. In two cases, the RU occurred in a healthy uterus and during labour, i.e. a percentage of 40%.

**1.9.3. Medium-term prognosis**

**1.9.3.1. Psychological complications :**

The experience of childbirth was judged to be bad or very bad in 60% of patients. The following psychological disorders were reported: extreme fatigue in 55% of cases, appetite problems in 22% and aggressiveness in 15% **(Table XXII).** In our study series, 21.7% of patients reported difficulty in caring for their babies.

**Table XXII: Medium-term prognosis**

| Psychological complications%. | |
|---|---|
| **Experience of childbirth** | |
| Very good | 15 .25 |
| Pretty good | 30 .51 |
| Mal | 25 .42 |
| Very bad | 28 .81 |
| **Psychological disorders** | |
| Extreme fatigue | 55 .93 |
| Aggressivity | 15 .25 |
| Behavioural disorder | 6,78 |

Appetite disorder22  .03

**Mother-baby relationship**

Excellent67  .24

Difficulty looking after your baby22  ,41

Feelings of anger and hatred towards your baby8  .62

Feeling guilty and unable to meet her baby's needs1  ,72

### 1.9.3.2. Sexual disorders

The patients in our series were asked about their sexuality. It turned out that :

■ The average time taken to return to sexual activity was 2.9 months.

■ Seventy reported a decrease in the frequency of sexual intercourse, with the fear of another pregnancy in 32% of cases and feelings of extreme tiredness hindering sexual fulfilment in 17%,

■ A reduction in libido was noted in 42.1% of cases, and 75.9% of patients said they had no desire to become pregnant again.

■ Although the majority of women interviewed stated that they were not considering a new pregnancy, 18 pregnancies were recorded and the average inter-genetic interval was 2.01.

## 2. Analytical study

### 2.1. Comparison of epidemiological characteristics and risk factors between healthy and scarred uterus

The median parity of patients in the scar uterus group was significantly higher than that in the healthy uterus group (p = 0.013).

We found a significantly higher mean BMI and freight macrosomia rate in the healthy uterus group than in the scar uterus group. **(Table XXIII).**

**Table XXIII: Comparison of epidemiological characteristics and risk factors between the healthy and scar uterus RU groups**

| Features | Healthy uterus | Scarred uteri | P |
|---|---|---|---|
| Average age of patients | 30,80 ± 2,083 | 30,89 ± 0,672 | 0.658 |
| Average gestational age | 40,3±0.62 | 39.19±0.22 | 0.164 |
| Parite | 3.6±0.51 | 2.47±0.089 | **0.013** |
| BMI | 34,55 ± 3,03 | 28,43 ± 0,57 | **0.033** |
| Macrosomia: Weight > 4 kg | 60% | 16% | **0.018** |
| Hydramnios (N) | 0 | 2 | 0.66 |
| History of myomectomy | 0 | 7(12.72%) | 0.4 |
| Multiple pregnancy | 0 | 2(3.36%) | 0.66 |
| Boundary basin | 1(20%) | 8(14.54%) | 0.74 |
| Dystocic presentation | 0 | 12,2% | 0.80 |

## 2.2. Comparison of UC types between healthy uterus and scar uterus groups

We found a significant difference in the type of lesion (complete or incomplete) between the two groups, with 65.5% of UC incomplete in the scar group compared with 20% in the healthy group (p=0.045) **(Figure 10).**

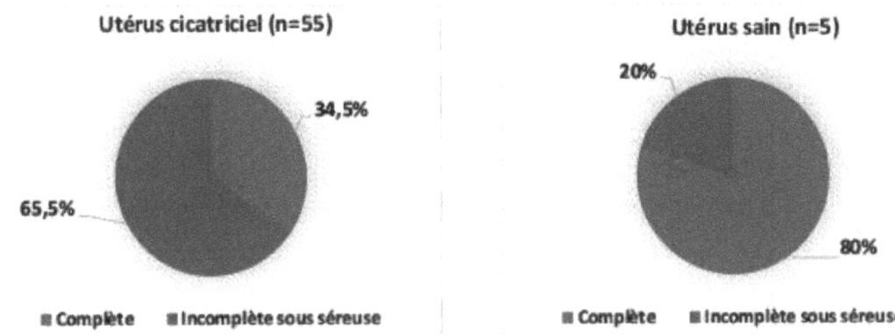


Figure 10. Distribution of UC according to lesion type.

## 2.3. Comparison of the characteristics of work and delivery between the healthy uterus and uterus groups scar

We found a significant difference in the onset of labour between healthy and scarred uteri (p=0.043).

Similarly, the duration of the active phase was significantly shorter in the healthy uterus group than in the scar uterus group **(Table XXIV).**

**Table XXIV: Comparison of labour and delivery characteristics between the healthy uterus and scar uterus groups**

| Features | Healthy uterus | Scarred uteri | P |
|---|---|---|---|
| Starting work | 80% | 20% | **0.043** |
| Oxytocin infusion | 60% | 0,0 | - |
| Dystocic presentation | 0 | 12,2% | 0,425 |
| Average duration of active phase (hours) | 0.57 ±0.2 | 2.86 ±0.54 | **0.000** |
| Instrumental delivery | 0 | 3.6% | 0.66 |
| Cesarean section | 60% | 90% | 0.518 |
| RCF abnormality | 40% | 52,7% | 0.596 |
| Uterine hypercinesia | 0 | 9% | 0.48 |

## 2.4. Comparison of maternal and fetal prognostic factors between the healthy uterus and scar uterus groups

The maternal complications studied were significantly more frequent in the case of RU on a healthy uterus.

In the scar uterus group, the fatal prognosis was less severe. In fact, in 75% of RU in scar uteruses, the Apgar score was greater than 7 compared with only 20% in the healthy uterus group. The difference was statistically significant at p=0.011 **(Table XXV).**

**Table XXV: Comparison of maternal and fetal prognostic factors between groups: healthy and scarred uterus**

| Features | Healthy uterus % | Scarred uteri % | P |
|---|---|---|---|
| Post-partum haemorrhage | 60,0 | 14,5 | **0.039** |
| Hysterectomy | 40,0 | 3,6 | **0.032** |
| Blood transfusion | 60,0 | 20,0 | **0,009** |
| Hospital stay > 5 days | 80,0 | 25,4 | **0.025** |
| APGAR score < 7 | 80,0 | 24,5 | **0.011** |

## 2.5. Analysis of the distribution of the anatomical location of uterine rupture

### 2.5.1. Between the healthy uterus and scar uterus groups

Among the 55 cases of scar uterus, the site of rupture was corporal or corporal-segmental in 12 cases, i.e. 21.8%. In contrast, this rate was 100% in cases of healthy uterus and the difference was statistically significant.

Vaginal and cervical lesions were statistically more frequent in cases of healthy uterus (**Table XXVI**).

**Table XXVI. Comparison of anatomical characteristics of the RU between healthy and scarred uterus**

| RU headquarters | Healthy uterus | Scarred uterus % (%) | P |
|---|---|---|---|
| Segment | 0 | 78.2 | n nnn |
| Body | 100 | 21.8 | |
| Cervical lesion | 60 | 3.63 | **0,003** |
| Vaginal lesion | 80 | 0 | **0.000** |
| Bladder lesion | 20 | 9 | 0.099 |

### 2.5.2. Between complete rupture and incomplete rupture

Of the 37 incomplete UCs, 33 were segmental. Conversely, out of 23 complete UCs, only 10 were segmental. Hence there was a significant relationship between the seat and the type of UC (p=0.0001) **(Table XXIV)**.

### 2.5.3. Depending on the moment of discovery

Among the 10 cases of RU before labour, 4 cases of RU were physical, i.e. 40%. Conversely, among the 50 cases of rupture that occurred during labour, the site of the rupture was corporal in only 13 cases, i.e. 26%. However, the difference was statistically insignificant (p=0.86) **(table XXVII)**.

**Table XXVII: Breakdown of the RU headquarters according to the type of break and the time of discovery.**

| RU locations | Complete | Incomplete | Before work | During work |
|---|---|---|---|---|

| | N | % | N | % | N | % | N | % |
|---|---|---|---|---|---|---|---|---|
| Segment | 10 | 43,5 | 33 | 89,2 | | 660,0 | 37 | 74,0 |
| Corporeal | 13 | 56,5 | 4 | 10,8 | | 440,0 | 13 | 26,0 |
| **Value of p** | | 0.0001 | | | | | 0.84 | |

**Table XVIII** summarises the comparative study between the two groups: healthy uterus and scar uterus. A significant difference was found in the type of rupture, its location and maternal-fetal complications. The mean parity, mean BMI and fatal weight were significantly higher in the healthy uterus group (**Table XVIII**).

### Table XXIX: Comparison of epidemiological, clinical , anatomical and prognostic characteristics of UR between healthy and scarred uterus

| Features | Healthy uterus N=5 | Scarred uteri N=55 | P |
|---|---|---|---|
| Medium parity | 3.6+0.51 | 2.47+0.089 | **0.013** |
| Average BMI | 34,55± 3,03 | 28,43 ± 0,57 | **0.033** |
| Macrosomia (weight>4kg) | 60% | 16% | **0.018** |
| Type of uterine rupture | | | |
| Incomplete break | 1(20%) | 36(65,5%) | **0.045** |
| Complete break | 4(80%) | 19(34,5%) | |
| Starting work | 80% | 20% | **0.043** |
| Average length of active phase | 0.57 + 0.2 | 2.86 + 0.54 | **0.000** |
| Maternal and fatal complications | | | |
| Post-partum haemorrhage | 60% | 14,5% | **0.039** |
| Hysterectomy | 40% | 3,6% | **0.032** |
| Blood transfusion | 60% | 20,0% | **0,009** |
| Hospital stay >5 days | 80% | 25,4% | **0.025** |
| APGAR score <7 | 80% | 24,5% | **0.001** |
| RU headquarters | | | |
| Segment | 0 | 78,2% | **0.00** |
| Corporeal | 100% | 21,8% | |
| Cervical lesion | 60% | 3.63% | **0.003** |
| Vaginal lesion | 80% | 0 | **0.00** |

## 1. Epidemiology of uterine rupture

### 1.1. Frequency of uterine rupture

In our series we recorded a rate of uterine rupture of 2.1^. This rate is among the highest of the Tunisian series (**Table XXVIII**). In fact, the frequency of RU varied between 0.86^ at the Sfax maternity centre and 2.69^ at our maternity hospital during the period 1989-1993.

**Table XXVIII: Frequency of UR in Tunisian series**

| Author | Hospital | Period | Workforce | Frequency (‰) |
|---|---|---|---|---|
| Kamoun [8] | Sfax | 1986-1991 | 40 | 0.86 |
| Arfaoui [9] | Menzel Bourguiba | 1986-1993 | 30 | 1.48 |
| Marouni [10] | CMNM | 1989-1993 | 51 | 2.69 |
| Ferchichi [11] | Rabta-Tunis | 1996-2000 | 41 | 1.38 |
| Attaya [12] | Nabeul | 1997-2003 | 35 | 1.3 |
| Hammami [13] | Military Tunis | 1992-2003 | 38 | 1.35 |
| Our series | CMNM | 2017-2021 | 60 | 2.1 |

The rates of UR in national series are intermediate between those observed in developed countries **(Table XXIX)** and those observed in underdeveloped countries, especially in Africa **(Table XXX). In fact,** UR is a very rare event in medicalised countries, with rates as low as 2/10000 in the United Kingdom [14] and 1.6/100000 in Italy [15].

**Table XXIX: Frequency of UC in developed countries**

| | Country | Period | Frequency |
|---|---|---|---|
| Zwart et al [16] | Netherlands | 2004-2005 | 5.9/10.000 |
| Fitzpatrick [14] | United Kingdom | 2009-2010 | 2/10.000 |
| Vanden Berghe [2] | Belgium | 2012-2013 | 3.6/10.000 |
| Donati [15] | Italy | 2014-2016 | 1.6/10.000 |
| Figueiro Filho [17] | Canada | 1998-2017 | 0.1% |
| Chang [18] | New Zelande | 2008-2018 | 8.1/10.000 |
| Wan et all [19] | China | 2013-2020 | 1.96/10.000 |

These rates are much higher in under-medicalised countries, where frightening figures of around 16% are reached, as is the case in Ethiopia [20], i.e. 1,000 times the frequency found in Italy [15] **(Table XXX)**.

**Table XXX: Frequency of UC in under-medicalised countries**

| Author | Hospital | Period | Frequency [%] |
|---|---|---|---|
| Lankoande [21] | Burkina Faso | 1995 | 10.5 |
| Vangeenderhuysen [22] | Niger | 2002 | 2.2 |
| Gueye et all [23] | Senegal | 2013-2015 | 0.58 |

| Getahun [20] | Ethiopia | 2013-2017 | 16.68 |
| Balde et all [24] | Guinee | 2017-2020 | 0.44 |

Thus, it is clear that the frequency of UR depends on the level of social and health development, the quality of obstetric care and varies with the geographical area to which the population belongs. In addition, the variability of the reported incidence rates is explained by the heterogeneity of the definition of UR within the series, some having excluded incomplete or dehiscent UR.

### 1.1.1 Frequency of UR in a scarred uterus

In our series, 91.7% of all URs occurred in a scar uterus. This rate is among the highest in the national literature. In fact, the proportion of scar uterus cases in Tunisia varies from 45 to 68%.

**Table XXXI: Frequency of scarring of the uterus among UK women (national series).**

| Author | Period | Workforce | Frequency (%) |
|---|---|---|---|
| Kamoun[8] | 1987-1991 | 4045,0 | |
| Arfaoui[9] | 1986-1993 | 3046,6 | |
| Ferchichi[11] | 1996-2000 | 4158,5 | |
| Attaya[12] | 1997-2003 | 2468 | |
| **Our series** | 2007-2021 | 55 | 91,7% |

In developed countries, the proportion of scarred uterus among UC varies between 70 and 90% [14]. In contrast, these frequencies are relatively lower in black Africa, ranging from 12 to 41% [20]. This finding cannot be explained by the rarity of this complication in a scar uterus, but rather by the greater frequency of RU in healthy uteruses exhausted by repeated pregnancies under poor management conditions.

### 1.1.2 Frequency of RU in a healthy uterus

In underdeveloped countries, the incidence of RU in a healthy uterus is 1/287 for Abioudun in Nigeria [25] and 1/519 for Elkady in Egypt [26]. Ahmadi [27] in Tunisia found a rate of 1/2158. In our series this rate is 1.7 per 10,000.

In contrast, this rate is very low in developed countries, reaching frequencies of less than 1 per 10,000 [4]. In a recent registry study in Norway, Al zirqi found a rate of 3.26 per 100,000 [28].

### 1.2. Age of patients

The average maternal age was 30.88±0.635 with a peak between 26 and 30 years, which is consistent with certain national series (**Table XXXII**). In fact, Arfaoui found that URs were mainly of interest in the 21-30 age group, i.e. 78.57% of cases. This is also the case for Filho [17] and Zhan [29], who also found a higher risk of UR in women aged over 30.

**Table XXXII: Breakdown of UK by age (national series)**

| Age of patients<br>Authors | 21-30 % | 31-40 % | 41-50 % |
| --- | --- | --- | --- |
| Attaya [12] | 34,2 | 62,85 | 2,8 |
| Ferchichi [11] | 43,8 | 51,1 | 4,8 |
| Arfaoui [9] | 78,57 | 21,42 | 0 |
| Hammami [13] | 57,9 | 42,1 | 0 |
| Metteli [30] | 50 | 43,35 | 6,65 |
| **Our series** | **46,0** | **48,0** | **3** |

On the other hand, some authors report a maximum of RU for women under the age of 30, as is the case in African countries [31], [32].

These findings may be contributed to the socio-cultural environment in these countries encouraging women to marry at a very early age. This is an alarming sign because it means that women could lose not only their fertility but also their lives sooner.

## 1.3. Socio-economic conditions and pregnancy follow-up

Of our patients, 40% had a rural background and 31.66% did not monitor their pregnancies well. These high figures reflect the relationship between socio-economic conditions, the quality of follow-up and the incidence of UR during pregnancy.

Inadequate medical surveillance and low levels of health have a negative impact on the incidence of UC. This is the case in African countries, where 60% to 70% of cases of UC occur in women from disadvantaged backgrounds [23].

Among our patients, taking into account the standards imposed by the national perinatal programme (4 prenatal consultations), we noted that only 40% of women who presented with an UR were correctly monitored in the healthy uterus group, compared with 69.1% in the scar uterus group. These inadequate pregnancy follow-up rates encourage us to improve the quality of follow-up, especially in the case of high-risk pregnancies such as scar uterus.

## 1.4. Risk factors

They are many and often interrelated:

### 1.4.1. The scarred uterus

A scarred uterus is a major risk factor for uterine rupture [17], [33] and [14]. On the other hand, a history of vaginal delivery appears to be a protective factor against RU [34].

#### 1.4.1.1 History of body scarring

The AHRQ considers that the risk of UC is increased when the scar is corporal [35], and therefore constitutes a contraindication to uterine testing according to the various learned societies in their recommendations for delivery in the case of a scarred uterus [36], [37] and [34]. Unfortunately, the frequency of scarring in our series was not determined due to lack of data.

### 1.4.1.2 : The number of uterine scars

Tahseen [38] has shown in a metanalysis that the risk of UC increases with the number of uterine scars, rising from 0.72% in the case of a single scar uterus to 1.59% in patients with 2 uterine scars. However, the authors are not unanimous. Indeed, some consider that the risk of UC is independent of the number of scars [39]. This is why the ACOG and the CNGOF authorise uterine testing in the case of bi-scarred uteri subject to a clear request from the patient and a favourable opinion from the medical team [36] and [34]. In our series, 9 cases of RU occurred in bi- or multi-scar uteri.

### 1.4.1.3 : Suturing technique

The suture technique is also important. Several authors explain that the risk of UR is greater when the uterine suture is made in a single plane [40].

### 1.4.1.4 : The uterine test

In a recent study in 2021, Filho [17] found an increased risk of RU in the event of uterine rupture. Several authors such as Macone [41] have tried to assess the probability of rupture in the event of uterine rupture by means of predictive scores in order to orientate the nature of the information and decide the route of delivery (**Table XXXIII**). In our series, the frequency of RU during a uterine test was 63%.

**Table XXXIII: Characteristics of the main predictive scores for the risk of uterine rupture [33].**

| Author [reference] Year of Publication, Type of study | Inclusion TVB/n (%) | Construction score validation | Factors predictive of risk of UR | Correlation : score-cesarean section score |
|---|---|---|---|---|
| Smith et al. 2005 Cohort retrospective 1985-2001 (N=23286) | 40-42 SA 100% TVB | - Construction of the Score: 1/2 cohort+ - Validation internal: 1/2 cohort | - Maternal age -Origin ethnic - Antecedent of AVB - Gestational age: 40-42 SA - Trigger - Baby's sex | - Low risk : 36% (<20 % C) - High risk : 16.5% (> 40% C) |
| -Macone et al. 2006 Cohort retrospective Case-control 1996-2000 | 134 UK after ABAC (case) versus 665 VABC without UK | -No validation external | - Maternal age - Age gestational - Origin ethnic - Previous | - Ante factors partum: not prediction reliable (AUC = 0.67) - Factors in |

| | | | | |
|---|---|---|---|---|
| | | | stroke<br>- Trigger<br>- Expansion >3cm | onset of work: no reliable model (AUC= 0.7)<br>- Sensib. max=75%<br>- And false+=40 |
| -**Grobman et al. 2006**<br>- **Prospective cohort** 1999-2002 (N=11855) | >=37 SA<br>100% TVB | - Construction of the Score: 1/2 cohort+<br>- Internal validation: 1/2 cohort after randomisation | - Antecedent of AVB<br>- Triggering | - No prediction reliable (AUC< 60%) |

AUC: Area under the curve; AVB: vaginal delivery; C: cesarean section; EPF: estimated weight fetal; TVB: attempted vaginal delivery; VBAC: vaginal delivery after caesarean section; RU: uterine rupture.

Other authors such as Rozenberghe suggest measuring the thickness of the lower segment between 35 and 38 SA. Jastrow [42] affirms the strong association between this measurement and the risk of the occurrence of RU. The threshold value is 2 to 3.5 mm depending on the ultrasound methods and techniques used.

However, the variations between observers and its poor positive predictive value mean that it cannot be used in everyday life.

Assessment of the uterine scar by measurement of the lower segment in the first trimester has also been proposed by other authors such as Stirnemann. 99% of the uterine scar is visible and it can be classified into 4 anatomical types according to its appearance [43] (Figure 11).

Although it seems interesting, no study has evaluated the association between the thickness of the lower segment measured in the 1$^{ier}$ trimester and the risk of dehiscence or uterine rupture.

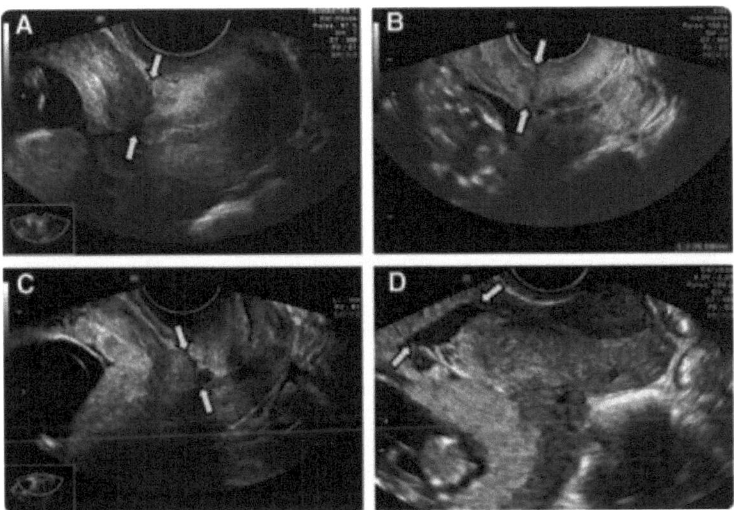

Figure 11. Endovaginal ultrasound of the cervico-isthmic defect in the 1st trimester of pregnancy. Example of a non-dehiscent and unexposed scar [A]; a non-dehiscent and exposed scar [B]; a dehiscent [>2mm wide] and unexposed scar [C]; a dehiscent [>2mm wide] exposed scar [type D] [54].

### 1.4.2. Previous uterine rupture

According to recent studies, the risk of recurrence of this complication varies between 0 and 35%, most often 9%. This depends on the type and location of the initial rupture [44]. Usta [45] in his study of 24 pregnancies after RU found 2 factors associated with recurrence of RU: a short time between pregnancies and the longitudinal nature of RU. However, Chibber [46] found cases of pregnancies, after conservative treatment of true UC, continued without recurrence.

In our series, none of the women had a history of uterine rupture.

### 1.4.3. Starting work

The onset of labour, whatever the technique used, is considered to be a risk factor in the presence or absence of uterine scarring [27]. Prostaglandin analogues multiply the risk of RU by 5.26 according to Traore [47] and by 4.9 according to Lyndon Rochelle [48]. The ACOG and HAS therefore recommend that they should not be used in a scarred uterus [36].

A 2016 meta-analysis by Lamourdediou [49] showed a risk of RU after cervical ripening by Foley catheter of 0.62%. For several authors, this method is the least likely to result in RU [50].

In addition, the use of oxytocin is considered by Landon MB [51] to have a high risk of the occurrence of RU, contrary to the results of Zelop [52] . The CNGOF does not contraindicate the reasoned use of oxytocin in spontaneous labour in a scar uterus [34].

Studies on healthy uteruses have also shown an increased risk of rupture when prostaglandin and oxytocin are used [53]. According to Sweeten [54], this is due to a lack of automated control of oxytocic infusion and systematic monitoring of labour.

In our series, 15 patients underwent labour induction: for scar uterus, induction was by AES in 5 cases and by detachment of the inferior pole of the uterus in 7 cases. The use of prostaglandins and oxytocics is contraindicated in cases of scar uterus in our department. In cases of RU in a healthy uterus, oxytocics were used in 60% of cases.

### 1.4.4. Multiparity

Multiparity is generally considered to be a risk factor for the development of RU through histological changes in the uterine muscle [55], [56]. Indeed, several authors consider that the risk of UC increases with parity [3], [17]. However, the proportion of multiparity in the incidence of UR varies greatly from one study to another **(Table XXXIV)**.

**Table XXXIV: Frequency of multiparity in the UK according to the literature**

| Author | Country | Period | Rate % (%) |
|---|---|---|---|
| Attaya [12] | Tunisia (Nabeul) | 1997-2003 | 28.5 |
| Ferchichi [11] | Tunisia (Tunis) | 1996-2000 | 38.8 |
| Rekik [57] | Tunisia (Sfax) | 1980-1984 | 41.4 |
| Metteli [30] | Tunisia (Bizerte) | 1987-1992 | 71 |
| Rahmen [58] | Morocco | 1985 | 83 |
| Mukasa [59] | Uganda | 2005-2006 | 38 |
| Delafield [60] | Mali | 2007-2008 | 46 |
| Donati [15] | Italy | 2014-2016 | 82.4 |
| **Our series** | CMNM | 2017-2021 | 1 |

This variability in the frequencies recorded is explained by the variation in the rates of multiparous women in the general population, other risk factors and, above all, the presence of a uterine scar. It is essentially the former Tunisian series and the African countries which have the highest proportions of multiparous women, due to the absence of a birth planning policy.

In our series, the multiparity factor only materialised in the healthy uterus group with a rate of 60%, whereas in the case of the scarred uterus, multiparous women represented only 5.5%. This could be explained by the fact that multiparity and uterine scarring are two independent risk factors.

### 1.4.5. Prolonged gestational age

Kiran [61] reported a higher risk of Ru after 40 days' amenorrhea, while Zelop found no significant difference between Ru before and after 40 days' amenorrhea. In our series, 25% of women had a term greater than 41 days' gestation.

### 1.4.6. Intergenic interval

Fitzpatrick [14] considers that there is an increased risk of UPR if the inter-genetic interval is less than 12 months. The ACOG recommends that patients who give birth within 18 to 24 months should be informed of the risk of developing RU [36]. The mean intergenic interval in our series was 13.4 months with extremes ranging from 4 months to 5 years.

### 1.4.7. Gynecological uterine scars

They are generally stronger than the obstetric scar. In the presence of a myomectomy scar, the non-opening of the uterine cavity is a criterion of solidity. Yaron Gil [62] in 2020 found a risk of UHR in the presence of myomectomy of 0.43%. Similarly, a review of the literature in 2015 showed that operative hysteroscopy is likely to leave uterine scars that may be detrimental to rupture [63]. In our series we found a history of myomectomy in 7 cases.

### 1.4.8. Endo-uterine manoeuvre

Endo uterine manoeuvres such as aspirations for termination of pregnancy or uterine revisions are considered to be factors in uterine fragility [64] and [54]. Such antecedents do not contraindicate vaginal delivery but uterine testing should be cautious [36] and [34]. In our series, 3 patients had a history of uterine revision and 10 others had a history of aspiration for termination of pregnancy.

### 1.4.9. Uterine distension

- **Macrosomia**: The data from studies is controversial. El kousy reported a higher risk of RU if the fatal weight exceeded 4kg [65]. Other authors such as Zelop and Guyot found no significant difference in the risk of rupture in the presence of fatal macrosomia [52].

Thus, for the RCOG [66], fatal weight in excess of 4 kg is a risk factor for rupture. On the other hand, ACOG and SOGC [67] and [68] did not find an association between fatal weight and the risk of this complication. In our series, Ona found a macrosomia rate of 16%.

- **Gemellaritis**: For some authors, uterine over-distension in the case of gemellaritis is not a factor in scar fragility [69]. Others do not recommend uterine testing in the case of multiple pregnancy, given the increased risk associated with it [70]. In the series reported here, two gemellar pregnancies were noted.

- **Hydramnios**: Some authors consider the risk of UR in the case of hydramnios to be high [71]. However, others such as Venditelli [69] do not consider excess fluid to be a factor in UR and authorise uterine testing in this case.

### 1.4.10.      Obesite

Yao R [72], showed in a study in 2019 that obesity increases the risk of RU in the event of uterine testing. These results are similar to those of Filho [17]. The mean BMI of the patients in our series was 28.9 and 41% were obese.

### 1.4.11.      Fetal pelvic disproportion - Pelvic anomalies :

Bone dystocia is one of the major causes of RU. In our study we recorded 9 cases of pathological pelvis, a rate of 15%. This rate was 3% in the study by Attaya [12]. In fact, the subjective nature of the clinical examination and the lack of availability of radiological examinations of the pelvis could be at the origin of the lack of recognition of dystocic pelvises.

**- Vicious presentation:**

dystocic presentations increase the risk of UR [73].

In our series we noted 7 presentations other than cephalic, one of which was a transverse presentation. The frequency of these presentations is 20% in Picaud's series [74].

In its latest recommendations for 2020, the French college authorises uterine testing in the event of a siege presentation [75].

### 1.4.12.      Work flow anomalies

In a study carried out in Ethiopia in 2020, Mengesha found an association between the presence of dynamic dystocia and the occurrence of UR [76].

### 1.4.13.      Others :

-      **Placentation abnormalities :**

They occur mainly in the presence of a scarred uterus and are considered a risk factor for UR by several authors [77] and [14].

-      **Obstetric manoeuvres and instrumental delivery** :

Kamoun reports 2 cases of abdominal expression. Ahmadi in his series of RU on a healthy uterus reports a moriceau manoeuvre in 2 cases, a Jacquemier manoeuvre in 1 case, a forceps extraction in 3 cases and a version with a large seat extraction for a gemellar delivery. In our series we found two cases of instrumental extraction on a scarred uterus in the face of acute foetal distress.

-      **In utero exposure to Diethylbestrol** :

Some authors have found a higher risk of UR in a healthy uterus in patients exposed in utero to diethylbestrol due to uterine hypoplasia [78],

-      **Uterine malformation :**

We did not record any cases of uterine malformations.

In the literature, the series by Bruand [79] in 2020 and Fernandes in 2016 report rare cases of UR occurring in a malformed uterus during pregnancy.

## 2. Clinical study and circumstances of discovery
### 2.1 . RU before term
UC can occur at any gestational age, but mainly at the end of pregnancy and during labour, regardless of the presence or absence of a uterine scar [4], [16], [80] and [14].

In particular situations, cases of early UR may occur. They are often described in cases of medical termination of pregnancy in the 2nd trimester, scar pregnancy and horn pregnancy [81]. Fuchs et all [82] report a case of RU on a rudimentary horn at 18 SA.

In fact, this condition is very rare, serious and occurs mainly in the case of a scarred uterus. A recent series by Maymon et al [83] reported 12 cases of preterm RU associated in 83.3% with placental insertion anomalies.

Maternal and neonatal outcomes can be improved by recognising the risk factors and clinical and ultrasound signs, in order to make the diagnosis in the shortest possible time and ensure rapid surgical intervention.

In our series, five cases of RUontete occurred during the 3rd trimester, representing a frequency of 8.3% of cases of RU. All patients had a scar uterus. The rupture was segmental and complete in 3 cases and incomplete in 2 cases. Thus even a segmental uterine scar can rupture before term and outside labour. Of course, there are two factors that can weaken the scar, namely placenta previa and hydramnios.

In other Tunisian series, Ferchichi [11] reported a case of RU in a woman with a uni-scarred uterus at 32 days' gestation for abnormally adherent placenta and hydramnios.

### 2.2 Uterine rupture at term (after 37 weeks' gestation)
In our series, RU was term in 91.7% of cases. Discovery was suspected either before the onset of labour, during labour or immediately post partum.

### 2.2.1 Discovery of UR during labour
RU was produced during labour in 87.2% of the total number of full-term RU and in 96% of cases of scar uterus. These results are consistent with the series by Zwart [16] in 2009, in which among 210 cases of UR 171 cases or 81.4% were produced during labour, of which: 73% occurred during the first stage of labour, 18.1% during the 2nd stage of labour and 8.8% during the latency phase. The mean gestational age was 40.2 SA. Other authors have similarly found a frequency of 75 to 80% of RU in a scarred uterus during a uterine test [14] and [84].

ECR abnormalities were the most frequently found signs in parturients (27/48). In the literature, these trace abnormalities are found in 55 to 90% of EC in a scar uterus [16], [85] independently of changes in uterine activity [86].

Persistent abdominopelvic pain despite analgesia or outside of contractions and of secondary onset should raise the alarm. It may be present in 50 to 70% of cases [16] and [14]. Metrorrhagia is a classic sign but is not constant [87]. Other signs may be associated with UR such as changes in uterine dynamics as described by Arulkumaran [88]. Given the absence of systematic monitoring of labour by tocography, we cannot determine the actual number of patients with this anomaly.

Similarly, failure to perceive the presentation is a common sign of uterine rupture [89].

UC in a healthy uterus presents heterogeneous and non-specific symptoms, leading to frequent delays in management and more serious complications. Installed metrorrhagia at the end of labour or in the immediate post-partum period should raise the alarm. In addition, some authors suggest that the symptoms are pain resistant to analgesia and unexplained maternal hypotension [27], [90], [91]. Wang [92] found in his series of RU on healthy uterus the presence of RCF abnormalities in 80% of cases.

In the Tunisian literature, many authors also consider that acute fetal distress is the first sign suggestive of this complication **(Table XXXV).**

**Table XXXV: Frequency of symptoms of UR during labour in the literature.**

| Author | Metrorragie | | SFA | | MDCU | | AD | | State of shock | |
|---|---|---|---|---|---|---|---|---|---|---|
| | NC | C | NC | C | NC | C | NCC | | NC | C |
| | % | % | % | % | % | % | % | % | % | % |
| Attaya [12] | 18,2 | 12,5 | 18,2 | 20,8 | - | - | 18,2 | 4,1 | 18,2 | 12,3 |
| Kaabar [93] | 44,4 | 29,0 | - | 21,0 | - | 19,2 | 44,4 | 31,0 | 55,5 | 8,7 |
| Metteli[30] | 28,5 | 9,0 | 57,1 | 12,0 | 14,3 | 4,0 | 14,28 | 4,0 | 28,6 | 4,0 |
| Ferchichi[11] | 23,5 | 33,3 | 29,4 | 29,0 | 11,7 | 37,5 | 35,2 | 25,0 | 11,7 | 8,3 |
| Arfaoui[9] | 31,2 | 35,7 | 43,7 | 50,0 | 12,5 | 7,14 | 12,5 | - | 18,7 | 35,7 |
| Our series | 40 | 18 | 40 | 50 | 0 | 10 | 0 | 6 | 20 | 4 |

Apart from one SFA, the frequencies reported in our study are either in the middle or among the lowest in the Tunisian literature.

This probably has to do with early diagnosis. The diagnosis of RU should not wait until a state of shock has set in. Emergency laparotomy is essential for the slightest suspicion of uterine rupture, particularly in the case of abnormalities of the fetal heart rate.

## 2.2.2. Discovery of RU before labour

RU was discovered outside labour in 7 cases out of 55, i.e. in 12.7%. It was a scar uterus in all cases. The discovery was fortuitous in 4 cases during a planned cesarean section for a bi-scarred uterus and in 3 cases during an emergency cesarean section for a pathological RCF in a patient with a uni-scarred uterus. Thus, even outside labour, an abnormal FHR should raise the suspicion of RU, especially if the uterus is scarred. Similarly, the presence of other risk factors such as the number of uterine scars (in our case, 4 cases of bi-scar uterus) may reveal the occurrence of RU.

### 2.2.3 Immediate post-partum discovery

RU was discovered post partum in 5 cases, i.e. in 10% of cases of RU occurring during labour, and 8% of the total number of cases of RU. Of the cases of UC in a scar uterus discovered post partum, 2 cases of UC were discovered following systematic uterine revision in the presence of a scar uterus.

In a North American series [94] reporting 347 cases of UC occurring during uterine testing, 11.5% were diagnosed post partum. However, systematic uterine revision is no longer recommended in the case of a scarred uterus [34],[91] and [95] except in the presence of signs suggestive of RU: haemorrhage, persistent pelvic pain with analgesia, and unexplained abnormality of RCF in the 2nd part of labour. Thus, the discovery of RU in the immediate post partum period is not exceptional [5].

## 3. Anatomical lesions :

### 3.1 Type of break :

Rupture was incomplete in 61.7% of cases, i.e. 65.5% of scar uteri and 20% of healthy uteri.

Thus, a significantly higher frequency of incomplete rupture was found in cases of scarred uterus. These results are consistent with those of the national series **(Table XXXVII).**

**Table XXXVI: Distribution of uterine ruptures according to the anatomical type of lesion (national series).**

| Period | Workforce | Scarred uterus | | Healthy uterus | |
|---|---|---|---|---|---|
| | | Complete % | Incomplete % | Complete % | Incomplete % |
| Kaabar [93] 1986-1989 | 77 | 17.5 | 82.5 | 70 | 30 |
| Metteli [30] 1987-1992 | 32 | 48 | 52 | 70.1 | 28 |
| Ferchichi [11] 1996-2000 | 41 | 8.3 | 91.6 | 17.6 | 82.3 |
| Attaya [12] 1997-2003 | 35 | 41.7 | 58.3 | 81.8 | 18.2 |
| **Our 2017-2021 series** | **60** | **34.5** | **65.5** | **80** | **20** |

In the literature, Guyot et al [96] found 36 cases of incomplete RU, 69.5% of which were incomplete, compared with 30.5% of complete RU, with an overall rate of complete RU of 0.4% in deliveries with a scar uterus and 0.5% in the case of uterine testing.

Other studies, however, mainly from African countries, have found higher rates of complete rupture [97], [32] due to a higher frequency of RU in a healthy uterus and a lack of monitoring of pregnancy and delivery.

### 3.2 . Breaking site

Most authors consider that the preferred site of UC is the lower segment [98], [59] and [99]. In our series, UC was segmental in 71.7% of cases. In Tunisian series, the proportion of segmental location varies between 40% and 78% (**Table XXXVII**).

**Table XXXVII: Distribution of uterine ruptures according to the anatomical site of the lesion in the literature.**

| Author | Year | Segment | Corporeal | Body segment |
|---|---|---|---|---|
| Kaabar [93] | 1986-99 | 67.5 | 7.8 | 24.7 |
| Njim[100] | 1982-88 | 40.62 | 28.1 | 31.3 |
| Metteli[30] | 1987-92 | 71.87 | 9.73 | 15.62 |
| Arfaoui[9] | 1986-93 | 63.3 | 3.3 | 33.3 |
| Marouni[10] | 1989-93 | 58.82 | 3.92 | - |
| Ferchichi[11] | 1996-00 | 78 | 2.4 | 21.9 |
| Attaya[12] | 1998-03 | 65.7 | 14.2 | 20 |
| Our series | 2017-21 | 71.7 | 23.3 | 5 |

Segmental location was found to be significantly more frequent in cases of scar uterus than in cases of non-scar uterus. Similarly, it was found that incomplete Ru was segmental.

These results are similar to those of NKwey et all [101] who found that most often uterine rupture is an incomplete rupture opposite a segmental scar.

In general, when UR appears before labour, it is corporal, whereas if it occurs during labour it is segmental [102].

### 3.3 Associated lesions

We found five cervical tears, three uterine pedicle lesions, 6 bladder sores and 4 vaginal lesions. Attaya, in a series of 35 cases, reported 5 cases of cervical tears, 2 cases of uterine pedicle lesions and one case of round ligament tearing [12]. In a series from Mali, Omar Traore noted 3 cases of bladder lesions, 28 cases of vascular lesions and one cervical lesion[73].he stated that 70% of bladder lesions in obstetrics occur concomitantly with uterine rupture. Pedicle lesions remain the most dreaded accident, occurring especially in cases of lateral extension of the rupture [97].

## 4. Therapeutic aspects of UR

As uterine rupture is an obstetric emergency, treatment must be carried out without delay, with pre-, per- and post-operative resuscitation to ensure correct hemostasis of the lesions.

### 4.1 Resuscitation measures

It is essential that this complication is managed in consultation with the intensive care team. The anaesthetist must manage the haemorrhage and perform anaesthesia for the fetal extraction at the same time [103]. The French College of Obstetricians and Gynaecologists recommends general anaesthesia with induction in rapid sequence in the event of serious obstetric haemorrhage and a fortiori in the event of rupture [104]. At the same time, vascular filling to compensate for hypovolemic shock is necessary while waiting for blood substitutes in accordance with the 2004 recommendations (1 unit of RGC/ 1 unit of FFP). This management, which should be carried out as early as possible, can be summarised as follows:

- Placement of two good-calibre venous approaches
- Oxygen therapy by mask (3 litres per minute),
- Rapid infusion of crystalloid or colloid solutes to compensate for volemic loss,
- Immediate order of compatible red blood cells.

Blood transfusion, although not without risk, is often necessary and the number of packed red blood cells reflects the severity of bleeding. In our series, 14 patients were transfused and the mean number of packed red blood cells was 3. In cases of severe bleeding, a hemostasis disorder develops, associated with disseminated intravascular coagulation (DIC). This was the case in 4 patients in our series. This defibrination syndrome due to the diffusion of thrombin in the circulation generates diffuse microthrombi and a haemorrhagic syndrome aggravated by reactive fibrinolysis.

As explained by Bollaert (105), treatment of this defibrinatory syndrome (DIC) is essentially based on :

- Fresh frozen plasma (FFP) at a dose of 10 to 15 ml/kg. FFP is the only product that provides protein S, factor C and factor Willebrand metalloprotease. FFP transfusion is indicated in DIC with a PT of less than 35-40%.
- Platelet transfusion is only indicated if the platelet count is below 50 g/L.
- In the case of fibrinogen, however, since the situation is one of consumption, the usual yield is reduced. There is therefore no proven indication for the use of fibrinogen in DIC.

For the 4 patients who developed hemostasis disorders, transfusion of fresh frozen plasma was sufficient to correct these disorders in all cases, with a favourable outcome.

## 4.2 Surgical treatment

For the vast majority of authors, laparotomy is essential for any suspected symptomatic UC [24]. This was the case for all the patients in our study. However, some authors opt for abstention in certain cases of RU under close surveillance during the first 24 hours. These are asymptomatic dehiscences discovered fortuitously during uterine revision and which do not require surgical repair given the absence of impact of a surgical procedure on the immediate risks [91] . The operation must imperatively take certain parameters into account: the age of the patient, her parity, the extent of the lesions, the risks for future pregnancies, the resources and above all the experience of the obstetrical team [5].

### 4.2.1. Radical surgery (hysterectomy)

Hysterectomy was the recommended treatment for UC until the 1980s. Nowadays, it is mainly indicated in cases where repair has failed or is impossible [89]. 6% of cases in our series underwent hysterectomy. This frequency varies according to the authors **(Table XXXIII)**.

Ours is one of the lowest. This may be explained by the rapidity of management and the need to preserve fertility in young women with low parity as soon as possible. For most authors, apart from its mutilating nature, hysterectomy for hemostasis is the most effective treatment for UR [106] . It represents the best therapeutic alternative in the absence of pregnancy desire.

Hysterectomies in our series were total in the case of healthy uterus, i.e. a rate of 3.3%, whereas they were subtotal in the case of scar uterus. This can probably be explained by the fact that the extent of the lesions in the case of a scar uterus is smaller, allowing subtotal hysterectomy. In the Tunisian series [11], [107], and [12], the frequency of total hysterectomy is higher: 4.8%, 18.75% and 17.1% respectively.

Total hysterectomy presents 3 major difficulties compared with subtotal hysterectomy: detachment of the prevesical peritoneum, dissection of the cervix due to pregnancy impregnation and hemostasis of the cervico-vaginal arteries [108].

### 4.2.2 Conservative surgery

Conservative treatment should be carried out when uterine repair is possible. It has the advantage of being easy and rapid and of preserving fertility [81].

[87]   . In our series, simple suturing was performed in 93% of cases. This rate is in line with the results of Guyot, Yap and Diaz [96], [109].

In the literature, the frequency of simple sutures varies between 5.3% and 100% **(Table XXXVIIII)**.

**Table XXXVIII: Distribution of UC according to surgical procedures performed**

| Authors | Country | Suture % | Hysterectomy % |
| --- | --- | --- | --- |
| Chamiso [110] | Ethiopia | 5,3 | 94,7 |
| Solton MH [111] | Saudi Arabia | 72,7 | 27,3 |
| Gombert [97] | Senegal | 5,7 | 94,3 |
| Boutaleb [112] | Morocco | 83 | 17 |
| Champault [113] | Cameroon | 53 | 47 |
| Bohoussoa [32] | Ivory Coast | 37,6 | 62,4 |
| Drobo A [114] | Mali | 84 | 16 |
| Ozdimir [115] | Turkish | 29,4 | 70,6 |
| Diallo FB [116] | Niger | 56 | 44 |
| Picaud [74] | Gabon | 53,6 | 46,4 |
| Guyot [96] | France | 100 | 0 |
| Yap [109] | United States | 90,5 | 9,5 |

Tubal ligation is performed in 15% of cases of conservative treatment, whereas in other Tunisian series the rate is 37.5% in the Drira series [107], 32.4% in the Attalah series [117] and 55% in the Kamoun series [8].

Of course, simple suture combined with tubal sterilisation has the advantage of a hemostatic procedure that is both easy and rapid, and helps to prevent the risk of recurrence, which some estimate at 4% to 19% in a subsequent pregnancy [81].

However, increasing medical requirements mean that tubal ligation is probably practised less and less. This is because the decision is taken in an emergency during the operation, without the couple being informed beforehand.

## 5. Prognosis

### 5.1 Maternal prognosis

### 5.1.1 Maternal mortality

Maternal mortality in our series was 0%. This testifies to the improvement in obstetric care and adequate technical facilities. These results are consistent with countries with a high socioeconomic level where mortality rates are low, such as the following studies: Chang in 2020: 0% [18]; and Zwart in 2010: 0% [16].

In the AHRQ report published in 2015, of the eight studies included, no maternal deaths were recorded among cases of UR [118].

However, other studies show that maternal mortality is not zero. This is the case in countries with low socio-health development, where rates of : 11.26% in the study carried out in Côte d'Ivoire by Abauleth [119], 14% in a study carried out in Burkina Faso by Lankoande [21] and 17.1% in the study carried out in Central Africa by Sepou [120].

Several authors estimate a greater risk of mortality when uterine rupture occurs in a healthy uterus [27] and [16].

This is probably due to the implausibility of the diagnosis, the delay in treatment and the extent of the lesions.

Today, huge efforts are being made all over the world to promote maternal health and reduce the mortality rate by acting on the risk factors. As a result, many countries such as France have succeeded in reducing maternal mortality from haemorrhage, a major complication of RU. The latest national survey report in France on maternal mortality between 2013-2015 showed a significant decrease in maternal mortality due to obstetric haemorrhage, with the mortality ratio falling from 1.6 to 1 between 2007 and 2015 [121].

**5.1.2: Maternal morbidity :**

Even if the prognosis is life-saving, UR is still fraught with a number of complications, mainly haemorrhagic and infectious.

**5.1.2.1.     Anemie**

Postoperative anaemia was found in 19 cases, a rate of 31.7%. However, the hemoglobin level cannot be used as a reflection of blood loss because patients are often transfused intraoperatively. In the literature, blood transfusion is required in 20-55% of cases [99].

**5.1.2.2.     Infection**

In our series, postoperative infectious complications were found in 3.3% of cases. These were wall infections. Some authors even report cases of postoperative peritonitis. This is the case of Taleb who reported 2 cases out of 67 RU.

**5.1.2.3.     Thromboembolic complications**

These complications are serious but rare, thanks to systematic prophylaxis in our centre. We have not reported any cases of this complication.

**5.1.2.4.     Surgical complications**

We noted seven bladder lesions in our study. In the literature, urological lesions are described in 4 to 6% of cases [122]. Other surgical complications have been reported with varying frequency: Taleb

[123] described two cases of vesico-vaginal fistulas and Rahman [58] in Morocco described 13 cases of urogenital fistulas among 96 cases of UR.

**5.1.2.5.     Psychological complications**

The quality of communication, respect for the woman's privacy and consideration of her experience of childbirth are important components in the management of any childbirth, even in obstetric emergencies [116]. As uterine rupture is associated with a high maternal mortality rate, it is a traumatic experience for some women.

In our series, 60% of the women had a poor experience of childbirth. Several psychological problems were reported: extreme fatigue, appetite problems, aggressiveness and behavioural problems. This may be explained by a failure to recognise the importance of psychological support for parturients in the face of a life-threatening situation. These results are consistent with a Tunisian survey carried out in Tunis maternity hospitals evaluating the satisfaction of parturients after childbirth [124].

**5.1.2.6.      fertility prognosis :**

According to the CNGOF 2012 recommendations on delivery in a scar uterus, there is no contraindication to a new pregnancy in women who have had a uterine rupture [125]. However, the woman must be informed of this risk. In our series, we recorded 18 pregnancies.

## 5.2 . Perinatal prognosis

### 5.2.1. Freight mortality

Perinatal mortality varies according to the series between 8.7 and 14% [16], [87], [126]. Chang found a rate of 16% comparable to the results of the INOSS study in 2019 [36]. Guise JM found a mortality rate of 8% in a literature review including 21 studies in 2020. In under-medicalised countries, perinatal mortality can reach 90-100% [23].

The fatal prognosis is different whether the uterus is healthy or scarred. In fact, in ruptures in a scar uterus the prognosis is less serious and the fatality rate varies from 0 to 20% [8].

A review of the literature revealed the frequency of perinatal mortality in a number of countries. All these results are shown in **Table XXXIX.**

**Table XXXIX: Rates of perinatal mortality among cases of UR in the literature**

| Author | Year | Country | Workforce | Mortality |
|---|---|---|---|---|
| Ferchichi [11] | 1996-2000 | Tunisia | 41 | 25 |
| Attaya [12] | 1997-2004 | Tunisia | 35 | 8,5 |
| Giuliano [87] | 1987-2009 | France | 52 | 13,6 |
| Sayed Ahmed [127] | 1993-2012 | Egypt | 49 | 12,2 |
| Donati [15] | 2014-2016 | Italy | 74 | 18.9 |
| Traore [73] | 2016-2017 | Mali | 98 | 54,1 |
| Chang [18] | 2008-2018 | New Zealand | 32 | 15,6 |

### 5.2.2. Freight morbidity

The fatal prognosis depends on when the rupture is discovered and how quickly it is managed. Fitzpatrick [14] found that 15% of non-decomposed neonates developed another major complication such as neonatal encephalopathy or respiratory distress. Neonatal asphyxia was present in 31% of cases in a study carried out in the Netherlands [16]. In our study, the morbidity rate (defined by an APGAR score of less than 7 at 5 minutes) was 0.3%. Attaya in [12] reported a perinatal morbidity rate of 2.9% and Kamoun in [8] showed that this rate was 20%.

## 6. Recommendations

The seriousness of uterine rupture means that measures must be taken to prevent its occurrence and improve the maternal-foetal prognosis:

■ Birth planning to reduce the number of voluntary terminations of pregnancy, a factor that weakens the uterine wall, and to avoid multiple pregnancies.

■ Health education: encouraging pregnant women to have regular check-ups on their pregnancies, while improving the quality of monitoring in order to detect risk factors for uterine rupture.

■ A system to control the transfer of parturients in order to avoid overloading second and third level maternity units with cases of abusive transfers, which can only reduce the vigilance of the obstetric team with regard to patients at risk of uterine rupture.

■ Raising awareness among medical and paramedical staff of the risks of RU, especially in first-line maternity units, to ensure that cases at risk of uterine rupture are transferred as quickly as possible.

■ A well-considered indication for the first caesarean section because it determines the woman's obstetrical prognosis

■ Abandonment of corporal cesarean section. A tubal ligation should be proposed if this is not the case.

■ Regular monitoring of the pregnancy and the progress of labour, especially in the case of a scarred uterus.

### 6.1. During pregnancy

■ All dystocies of maternal or ovarian origin must be detected before the pregnant woman goes into labour.

■ In the case of a scarred uterus, the operative report must be available and must specify: the indication for the anterior cesarean section, the location of the uterus, the type of uterus and the type of operation.
the hysterotomy (segmental or corporal), its type, the suture technique and the post-operative course.

■ A permanent indication for vaginal delivery must be recognised, and an iterative cesarean section must be performed in this case before the start of labour.

■ In the absence of an operative report, we need to question the patient in greater depth in order to clarify the circumstances of the birth and the operative aftermath.

■ Check the report of a myomectomy and question the patient more thoroughly so as not to overlook a fragile scar that the woman underestimates.

■ A prophylactic cesarean section should be indicated when there is more than one uterine scar.

■ Once the indications for prophylactic caesarean section have been ruled out, a uterine test is carried out subject to close monitoring of pregnancy and labour. A radiopelvic scan and fatal weight assessment in the $3^{ieme}$ trimester to ensure that there is no fatal macrosomia and that the pelvis is normal should be performed systematically.

## 6.2. During work

❖*Recommendations on healthy uterus*:

■ The partogram must be closely monitored to detect any abnormalities in labour.

■ Look for signs of dystocia, fetal-pelvic disproportion and assess the pelvis.

■ Untimely obstetric manoeuvres should no longer be seen. Oxytocin infusion must be automated.

■ Avoid vaginal interventions before complete dilatation.

■ Train obstetricians and midwives to recognise the signs of uterine rupture.

■ *Recommendations for scar uterus*

■ A woman with a scarred uterus must be operated in a suitable environment with a functional operating theatre.

■ The uterine test must be rigorously monitored, and fatal heart rate and uterine dynamics recorded by external tocography as a matter of course.

■ A uterine test must be interrupted at the slightest abnormality in labour.

o Any abdominal pain that is secondary in onset or unresponsive to analgesia may be a warning sign of uterine rupture.

■ Appropriate surgical techniques must be optimised during a cesarean section, and we recommend a double-layer suture to prevent the risk of UR, especially when the cesarean section is performed outside labour.

## 6.3. After childbirth

❖ Every woman undergoing caesarean section must have an operative report that includes the indication for the section, the type of incision and sutures and the postoperative history.

❖ All women should be educated about the need for effective contraception in order to space pregnancies, and informed about the risk of uterine rupture if a pregnancy occurs within 18 to 24 months.

## 7. Limitations and strengths of the study

- The weaknesses of our study are

♦ ♦♦ A retrospective analysis of the files. In fact, the data is often incomplete and certain parameters are not collected, such as the incision technique used during the previous cesarean section and the post-operative follow-up.

♦ ♦♦ The limited size of the sample, which complicates statistical analysis.

♦ ♦♦ The monocentric nature of the study

- Highlights:

♦♦♦ Our study constitutes the first of its kind in our department to study this pathology and to describe its epidemiological, clinical and prognostic characteristics in the presence or absence of a uterine scar.

♦♦♦ Among the strong points of our study was the multidimensional aspect which enabled us to answer the various questions relating to uterine rupture (epidemiological, therapeutic and prognostic aspects).

## 5 Conclusion

Uterine rupture is defined as complete or incomplete non-surgical termination of the body or lower segment of the pregnant uterus.

This is a serious hemorrhagic complication of childbirth that can seriously compromise the mother's vital prognosis, and can even be fatal.

It is rare, and its frequency is a good indicator of a country's level of medicalisation. Although it has become the exception in developed countries, it remains the prerogative of underdeveloped countries.

In Tunisia, it contributes to maternal mortality despite prevention efforts. Diagnosis is exclusively clinical, and treatment can be mutilating.

The aim of this study is to examine the epidemiological and clinical profile of uterine rupture, as well as the different therapeutic modalities and elements of maternal-fatal prognosis, in order to propose recommendations aimed at reducing the frequency of this complication in our country.

We conducted a retrospective, descriptive, single-centre, cross-sectional, analytical study at the Monastir maternity and neonatology centre over a 5-year period from 1 January 2017 to 31 December 2021.

We also carried out a retrospective survey of the patients included in our study to assess their experiences of childbirth and their sexuality at least 6 months after childbirth.

We included all patients with uterine rupture during the study period. A total of 60 cases were included. For each patient, we collected epidemiological data, gynaeco-obstetric antecedents and clinical data. We also reported on the positive diagnosis, therapeutic management and prognosis.

During this period, we recorded 28,546 deliveries and 9996 caesarean sections (35.1%). The rate of uterine rupture was 2.13^.

In 55 cases, uterine rupture occurred in a scar uterus, i.e. a frequency of 91.6%, of which 41 cases were patients with uni-scar uteri.

The mean age of the patients was 38.88 years, with extremes of 18 and 42 years, and 41.6% were obese. The mean parity was 2.57, with extremes ranging from 2 to 5. 60% of patients were of urban origin, and 31.6% of pregnancies were poorly monitored. Antecedent myomectomy was present in 7 scarred patients (11.6%). Five cases of rupture occurred before 37 SA, between 34 and 36. All patients had a scar uterus and the clinical sign of rupture was a pathological RCF in 4 cases. The rupture was segmental-corporeal and complete in 3 cases and incomplete segmental in 2 cases. The treatment was conservative surgery in 4 patients, and there was one case of hysterectomy for post-partum haemorrhage that refused medical treatment.

Of the 55 cases that occurred after 37 weeks' gestation, 40 patients, or 66.7% of the total number, were at term. Fourteen patients had a prolonged term and one was over term. The most common clinical sign was an abnormal FPR for cases in healthy and scar uterus. We noted 12.7% of ruptures outside labour, 4 of which were discovered incidentally during a planned cesarean section for a bi-scarred uterus.

The majority of cases of RU were discovered during labour, i.e. 78.1% of the total rate, and 71% of cases of RU in a scar uterus. Ruptures in a healthy uterus occurred after complete dilatation and post partum in 80% of cases. Labour was induced in 25% of the overall rate of RU and in 80% of RU in healthy uterus. . We noted 2 instrumental deliveries on a scar uterus for a declared RCF with complete dilatation and 48 patients delivered by emergency cesarean section.

UC was incomplete in 61.7% of cases. In contrast to the healthy uterus, the majority of UC in the scar uterus was incomplete, with frequencies of 20% and 65.5% respectively. The difference was statistically significant. The site of uterine rupture was corporal or segmental-corporeal in 28.3%. This location was involved in 21.8% of uterine ruptures in scar uterus and 100% of uterine ruptures in non-scar uterus. The difference was statistically significant.

The site of rupture was segmental in 89.2% of incomplete ruptures and 43.5% of complete uterine ruptures. The difference was statistically significant. Similarly, the seat was corporeal in 40% of uterine ruptures that occurred outside labour, compared with 26% of uterine ruptures that occurred during labour. However, the difference was not significant.

Lesions associated with uterine rupture were as follows: cervical lesions (8.3% of cases), lesions of the uterine pedicle (5% of cases), and vaginal lesions (6.7% of cases).

Conservative surgical treatment using simple sutures was performed in 93.3% of cases. Associated tubal ligation was performed in 15% of cases. Hysterectomy for hemostasis was necessary in 6% of patients, i.e. 3.6% of uterine ruptures in scar uterus and 40% of uterine ruptures in non-scar uterus.

Blood transfusion was used in 14 patients. The average number of packed red blood cells transfused was 3, with extremes of 2 to 6 packed red blood cells.

Maternal mortality was 0%. Intraoperative complications included haemorrhage in 11 cases and bladder injury in 6 cases.

We noted the following post-operative complications: anaemia in 31.7% of cases, urinary tract infection in 6.7% of cases and prolonged hospitalisation in 30% of cases.

Sixty patients had had a bad experience of childbirth. Psychological problems were represented by extreme fatigue in 55% of the patients questioned, an appetite problem in 22% of cases and aggressiveness in 15% of cases. The average time taken to resume sexual activity was 2.9 months.

In terms of fatality, the perinatal mortality rate was 11%. In 30% of cases we recorded an Apgar score of less than 7 at 5 minutes. The fatal prognosis was significantly less severe in cases of uterine rupture in a scar uterus.

At the end of this study, based on our experience and reviews of the literature, we proposed practical recommendations to reduce the incidence of this obstetric complication in our country.

At the end of this work, we can conclude that uterine rupture is a potentially serious pathology that can be life-threatening or fatal. Early diagnosis is essential for appropriate management.

# 6 References


1.   Fox NS, Gerber RS, Mourad M et al. Pregnancy outcomes in patients with prior uterine rupture or dehiscence. Obstet Gynecol 2014; 123: 785-789.

2.   Vandenberghe G, De Blaere M, Van Leeuw V, Roelens K, Englert Y, Hanssens M, et al. Nationwide population-based cohort study of uterine rupture in Belgium: results from the Belgian Obstetric Surveillance System. BMJ Open. May 2016;6(5):e010415.

3.   Al-Zirqi I, Daltveit AK, Forsen L, Stray-Pedersen B, Vangen S. Risk factors for complete uterine rupture. Am J Obstet Gynecol. Feb2017; 216(2):165.e1-165.e8.

4.   Hofmeyr GJ, Say L, Gulmezoglu AM. WHO systematic review of maternal mortality and morbidity: the prevalence of uterine rupture. BJOG IntJ Obstet Gynaecol. Sept 2005; 112(9) :1221-8.

5.   Fatfouta I, Villeroy de Galhau S, Dietsch J, Eicher E, Perrin D. Spontaneous uterine rupture in a healthy uterus during labour: a case report and review of the literature. J Gynecologie Obstetrique Biol Reprod. Apr 2008;37(2):200-3.

6.   tej dellagi. Tej Dellagi Rafla, Bougatef Souha, Ben Salah Faygal, Ben Mansour Nadia, Gzara Ahlem, Gritli Ibtissem, Ben Romdhane H, Rachdi MT. l 'enquete nationale tunisienne sur la mortalite maternelle de 2010: a propos des données de Tunis. La Tunisie Medicale - 2014; Vol 92 (n°08): 560-566.

7.   MICS 4 Multiple Indicator Cluster Survey (2011-2012).

8.   Kamoun M. Les ruptures uterines a la maternite de Sfax. These Medecine Sfax 1994: 40.

9.   Arfaoui F. les ruptures uterines a propos de 30 cas a la maternite de l'hopital Menzel Bourguiba de janvier 1986a decembre 1993.These Medecine Tunis 1994 :201.

10. Marouni S. Les ruptures uterines a propos de 51 cas vus a la maternite de Monastir. These Medecine Monastir 1995: 261.

11. Ferchichi Nabil. Rupture uterine a propos de 41 cas su service A du centre de maternite et de neonatologie de la Rabta. These medecine Tunis 2001:102.

12. Attaya S. Uterine rupture: epidemiology, prognosis and treatment (About 35 cases). These Med Monastir 2005 TH/MO1364.

13. Hammami F. les ruptures uterines propos de 38 cas. Experience de la maternite de l'hopital militaire de tunis.2004 :319.

14. Fitzpatrick KE, Kurinczuk JJ, Alfirevic Z, Spark P, Brocklehurst P, Knight M. Uterine rupture by intended mode of delivery in the UK: a national case-control study. PLoS Med. 2012;9(3): e1001184.

15. Donati S, Fano V, Maraschini A. Uterine rupture: Results from a prospective population-based study in Italy. Eur J Obstet Gynecol Reprod Biol. Sept 2021; 264:70-5.

16. Zwart JJ, Richters JM, Ory F, de Vries JIP, Bloemenkamp KWM, van Roosmalen J. Uterine rupture in The Netherlands: a nationwide population-based cohort study. BJOG Int'J Obstet Gynaecol. Jul 2009;116(8):1069-78; discussion 1078-1080.

17. Figueiro-Filho EA, Gomez JM, Farine D. Risk Factors Associated with Uterine Rupture and Dehiscence: A Cross-Sectional Canadian Study. Rev Bras Ginecol E Obstetricia RBGO Gynecol Obstet. Nov 2021;43(11):820-5.

18. Chang Y. Uterine rupture over 11 years: A retrospective descriptive study. Aust N Z J Obstet Gynaecol. Oct 2020;60(5):709-13.

19. Wan S, Yang M, Pei J, Zhao X, Zhou C, Wu Y, et al. Pregnancy outcomes and associated factors for uterine rupture: an 8 years population-based retrospective study. BMC Pregnancy Childbirth. Dec 2022;22(1):91.

20. Getahun WT, Solomon AA, Kassie FY, Kasaye HK, Denekew HT. Uterine rupture among mothers admitted for obstetrics care and associated factors in referral hospitals of Amhara regional state, institution-based cross-sectional study, Northern Ethiopia, 2013-2017. PloS One. 2018 ;13(12): e0208470.

21. Lankoande J, Oijedraogo C, Toure B, Ouedraogo A, Dao B, Kone B. Les ruptures uterines obstetricales a la maternite du centre hospitalier national de Ouagadougou: A propos de 80 cas colliges en une annee d'activite obstetricale.1998 [cite 10 aout 2022];

22. Vangeenderhuysen C, Souidi A. Rupture uterine sur uterus gravide: étude d'une serie continue de 63 cas a la maternite de référence de Niamey (Niger). Medecine Trop Rev Corps Sante Colon. 2002 ;62(6):615-8.

23. Gueye I, thiam m, niang m, sarr fr, ba p, mahamat s, et al. Ruptures uterines a l'hopital regional de Thies (Senegal). j sago. 1 jan 2016; 17:28-32.

24. Balde IS, Sylla I, Diallo MH, Diallo IT, Diallo FB, II Sow A, et al. Evolution des Ruptures Uterines a la Maternite de L'hopital National Ignace Deen (Chu de Conakry). Medecine Trop Sante Int. 29 Jan 2021 ;1(1):ZY14-QG95.

25. Abiodun P. A, Ijaiya MDA, Yahaya UR. Ruptured Uterus: A Study of 100 Consecutive Cases in Ilorin, Nigeria. J Obstet Gynaecol Res. Dec 2001;27(6):341-8.

26. Elkady AA. Elkady AA, Bayomy HM, Bekhiet MT, Nagib HS, Wahba AK. A review of 126 cases of ruptured gravid uterus. Int Surg 1993;78(3):231-5.

27. Ahmadi S, Nouira M, Bibi M, Bouguizane S, Saidi H, Chaib A, et al. Uterine rupture in healthy pregnant uterus. A propos de 28 cas. Gynecologie Obstetrique Fertil. Sept 2003 ;31(9):713-7.

28. Al-Zirqi I, Daltveit AK, Vangen S. Infant outcome after complete uterine rupture. Am J Obstet Gynecol. Jul 2018;219(1): 109.e1-109.e8.

29. Zhan W, Zhu J, Hua X, Ye J, Chen Q, Zhang J. Epidemiology of uterine rupture among pregnant women in China and development of a risk prediction model: analysis of data from a multicenter, cross-sectional study. BMJ Open. 29 Nov 2021;11(11): e054540.

30. Metteli MS. Contribution a l'etude des ruptures uterines sur une periode de 5 ans a la maternite de Bizerte a propos de 32 cas. These Med. Tunis1992:201.

31. Bayo A Les ruptures uterines a propos de 58 cas recenses a l'hopital Gabriel Toure. These de Medecine, Bamako, 1991, No1.

32. Bohoussou K, Houphouet K.B., Anoma M. Sangaret M. A. Uterine rupture during labour. A propos de 128 cas Afr.Med. 1978, 17, (162), 467-478.

33. Parant O. Uterine rupture: prediction, diagnosis and management. J Gynecologie Obstetrique Biol Reprod. dec 2012;41(8):803-16.

34. Carbonne, B., Frydman, R., Goffinet, F., Pierre, F., Subtil, D., d'Ercole, C. Truffert, P. (2000). Recommandations pour la pratique clinique : cesarienne consequences et indications. CNGOF; 2000.

35. Agency for Healthcare Research and Quality. Vaginal birth after cesarean: new

insights. AHRQ Publication No. 10-E003 2010.

36. ACOG Practice Bulletin No. 205: Vaginal Birth After Cesarean Delivery. Obstet Gynecol. February 2019;133(2): e110-27.

37. Royal College of Obstetricians and Gynecologists. Birth after previous Caesarian birth. Green-Top Guideline, 2007 (www.rcog.org.uk).

38. Tahseen S, Griffiths M. Vaginal birth after two caesarean sections (VBAC-2)-a systematic review with meta-analysis of success rate and adverse outcomes of VBAC-2 versus VBAC-1 and repeat (third) caesarean sections. BJOG. 2010;117(01):5-19. Doi: 10.1111/j.1471-0528.2009.02351.x.

39. Clark SL. Rupture Of scarred uterus. Obstet Gynecol Clin North Am 1988;15;4737- 45.

40. Roberge S, Demers S, Girard M, Vikhareva O, Markey S, Chaillet N, et al. Impact of uterine closure on residual myometrial thickness after cesarean: a randomized controlled trial. Am J Obstet Gynecol. Apr 2016;214(4): 507.e1-507.e6.

41. Macones GA, Cahill AG, Stamilio DM, Odibo A, Peipert J, Stevens EJ. Can uterine rupture in patients attempting vaginal birth after cesarean delivery be predicted? Am J Obstet Gynecol 2006; 195:1148-52.

42. Jastrow, N., et al, Sonographic lower uterine segment thickness and risk of uterine scar defect: a systematic review. J Obstet Gynaecol Can, 2010. 32(4): p. 321-7.

43. Stirnemann, J.J, et al, First-trimester uterine scar assessment by transvaginal ultrasound. Am J Obstet Gynecol, 2011. 205(6): p. 551 e1-6.

44. Lim AC, Kwee A, Bruinse HW. Pregnancy after uterine rupture: a report of5 cases and a review of the literature. Obstet Gynecol Surv 2005; 60:613-7.

45. Usta IM, Hamdi MA, Musa AA, Nassar AH. Pregnancy outcome in patients with previous uterine rupture. Acta Obstet Gynecol Scand 2007; 86:172-6.

46. Chibber R, El-Saleh E, Al Fadhli R, Al Jassar W, Al Harmi J. Uterine rupture and subsequent pregnancy outcome--how safe is it? A 25-year study. J Matern-Fetal Neonatal Med Off J Eur Assoc Perinat Med Fed Asia Ocean Perinat Soc Int Soc Perinat Obstet. May 2010;23(5):421-4.

47. Traore Y. Les ruptures uterines a l'hopital national du point G: facteurs influengant le pronostic materno foetal et mesures prophylactiques a propos de 180 cas. These de Medecine Bamako, 1996, n) 27.

48. Lydon-Rochelle M, Holt VL, Easterling TR, Martin DP. Risk of uterine rupture during labor among women with a prior cesarean delivery. N Engl J Med. 5 Jul 2001;345(1):3-8.

49. Lamourdedieu C, Gnisci A, Agostini A. Risk of uterine rupture after maturation of scar uteri by balloon catheter. J Gynecologie Obstetrique Biol Reprod. May 2016;45(5):496-501.

50. Ravasia DJ, Wood SL, Pollard JK. Uterine rupture during induced trial of labor among women with previous cesarean delivery. Am J Obstet Gynecol. Nov 2000;183(5):1176-9.

51. Landon MB, Grobman WA. What We Have Learned About Trial of Labor After Cesarean Delivery from the Maternal-Fetal Medicine Units Cesarean Registry. Semin Perinatol. August 2016;40(5):281 -6.

52. Zelop CM, Shipp TD, Cohen A, Repke JT, Lieberman E. Trial of labor after 40

weeks' gestation in women with prior cesarean section. Obstet Gynecol. March 2001;97(3):391-3.

53. Phuapradit W, Herabutya Y, Saropala N. Uterine rupture and labor induction with prostaglandins. J Med Assoc Thai 1993 May;76(5): 292-5.

54. Sweeten KM. Sweeten KM, Graves WK, Athanassiou A. Spontaneous rupture of the unscarred uterus. Am J Obstet Gynecol 1995;172(6):1851-5.

55. Kone M., Diarra S. Uterine rupture during pregnancy Encycl Med Chir(Paris-France),Obstetrique,5-080-A-10,1995:7.

56. Vilchez G, Nazeer S, Kumar K, Warren M, Dai J, Sokol RJ. Contemporary epidemiology and novel predictors of uterine rupture: a nationwide population-based study. Arch Gynecol Obstet. nov 2017;296(5):869-75.

57. Rekik S, Halouani L. Les ruptures uterines a la maternite de Sfax. A propos de 72 cas de 1980 a 1984. [Cite 30 aout 2022].

58. Rahman J, Al-Sibai MH, Rahman MS. Rupture of the uterus in labor. A review of 96 cases. Acta Obstet Gynecol Scand. 1985;64(4):311 -5.

59. Mukasa PK, Kabakyenga J, Senkungu JK, Ngonzi J, Kyalimpa M, Roosmalen VJ. Uterine rupture in a teaching hospital in Mbarara, western Uganda, unmatched case- control study. Reprod Health. 29 May 2013;10(1):29.

60. Delafield R, Pirkle CM, Dumont A. Predictors of uterine rupture in a large sample of women in Senegal and Mali: cross-sectional analysis of QUARITE trial data. BMC Pregnancy Childbirth. 1 Nov 2018;18(1):432.

61. Kiran TSU, Chui YK, Bethel J, Bhal PS. Is gestational age an independent variable affecting uterine scar rupture rates? Eur J Obstet Gynecol Reprod Biol. 1 May 2006;126(1):68-71.

62. Gil Y, Badeghiesh A, Suarthana E, Mansour F, Capmas P, Volodarsky-Perel A, et al. Risk of uterine rupture after myomectomy by laparoscopy or laparotomy. J Gynecol Obstet Hum Reprod. Oct 2020;49(8):101843.

63. Stankova T, Ganovska A, Stoianova M, Kovachev S. [Complications of diagnostic and operative hysteroscopy--Review]. Akush Ginekol (Sofiia). 2015;54(8):21-7.

64. Gibbins, K. J., Weber, T., Holmgren, C. M., Porter, T. F., Varner, M. W., & Manuck, T. A. (2015). Maternal and fetal morbidity associated with uterine rupture of the unscarred uterus. American journal of obstetrics and gynecology, 213(3), 382-e1.

65. Elkousy MA, Sammel M, Stevens E, Peipert JF, Macones G. The effect of birth weight on vaginal birth after cesarean delivery success rates. Am J Obstet Gynecol. March 2003;188(3):824-30.

66. Birth after previous caesarean birth. Rcog.org.uk. 2018. Available from: https://www.rcog.org.uk/globalassets/documents/guidelines/gtg_45.pdf [cited 4 November 2018]

67. American College of Obstetricians and Gynecologists 2010 (ACOG): www.acog.org.

68. Guidelines for vaginal birth after previous caesarean birth. Sogc.org. 2018. Available from: https://sogc.org/wpcontent/uploads/2013/01/155E-CPG-February2005.pdf. [cited 4 November 2018]

69. Vendittelli, j.l. tabaste, c.labarchede. vendittelli, j.l. tabaste, c.labarchede. Uterine rupture in a previously cesarised uterus. Review of the literature on two cases.

Rev.Fr Gynecol-Obstet, 1993, 88,5.

70. Coutty N, Deruelle P, Delahousse G, Legoueff F, Subtil D. Accouchement par voie basse des grossesses gemellaires sur uterus cicatriciel: peut-on autoriser l'epreuve uterine? Gynecologie Obstetrique Fertil. Oct 2004;32(10):855-9.

71. Zania R, Favier M.Uterus cicatriciels: la cesarienne iterative ne doit plus être systématique. Prat Med 1986,18:73-42.

72. Yao R, Crimmins SD, Contag SA, Kopelman JN, Goetzinger KR. Adverse perinatal outcomes associated with trial of labor after cesarean section at term in pregnancies complicated by maternal obesity. J Matern Fetal Neonatal Med. 18 Apr2019;32(8):1256-61.

73. Traore Soumana Oumar 1,Traore Alassane 2, Sylla Cheickna 3, Tall Saoudatou 1, , Doumbia Saleck 1, et al. Maternal-Fetal Prognosis of Uterine Rupture during Labour in the Commune V Health District of Bamako. Health Sci. Dis: Vol 21 (7) July 2020 pp 17-21 . [cited 13 august 2022].

74. Picaud A, Nlome-Nze AR, Ogowet N, Mouely G. Uterine rupture. Apropos of 31 cases seen at the Hospital Center of Libreville (Gabon). Rev Fr Gynecol Obstet. May 1989;84(5):411-6.

75. Azria E. Breech Presentation: CNGOF Guidelines for Clinical Practice - Case Selection for Trial of Labour. Gynecol Obstet Fertil Senol. Jan 2020;48(1):120-31.

76. Mengesha MB, Weldegeorges DA, Hailesilassie Y, Werid WM, Weldemariam MG, Welay FT, et al. Determinants of uterine rupture and its management outcomes among mothers who gave birth at public hospitals of Tigrai, North Ethiopia: an unmatched case control study. J Pregnancy. 2020; 2020:8878037. Doi: 10.1155/2020/8878037.

77. DeRoux SJ, Prendergast NC, Adsay NV. Spontaneous uterine rupture with fatal hemoperi- toneum due to placenta accreta percreta: a case report and review of the literature. Int J Gynecol Pathol 1999 Jan; 18(1):82-6.

78. Adams DM, Druzin ML, Cederqvist LL. Intrapartum uterine rupture. Obstet Gycol 1989;73:471-3.

79. Bruand M, Thubert T, Winer N, Gueudry P, Dochez V. Rupture of Noncommunicating Rudimentary Horn of Uterus at 12 Weeks' Gestation. Cureus. March 6, 2020;12(3):e7191.

80. Landon MB, Hauth JC, Leveno KJ, Spong CY, Leindecker S, Varner MW, et al. Maternal and perinatal outcomes associated with a trial of labor after prior cesarean delivery. N Engl J Med. 16 Dec 2004;351(25):2581-9.

81. Gautier C, VanBelle Y, VanBogaert LJ, DeMuylder. Gautier C, VanBelle Y, VanBogaert LJ, DeMuylder E. Rupture uterine: reflexion about a spontaneous case at mid-pregnancy. J Gycol Obstet Biol Reprod 1985 ;4:201-9.

82. Fuchs F, Guillot E, Cordier AG, Chis C, Raynal P, Panel P. Rupture of a rudimentary non-communicating uterine horn on a pseudo-unicorn uterus at 23 weeks of amenorrhoea. Gynecologie Obstetrique Fertil. avr2008;36(4):400-2.

83. Maymon R, Mor M, Betser M, Kugler N, Vaknin Z, Pekar-Zlotin M, et al. Second-trimester and early third-trimester spontaneous uterine rupture: A 32-year singlecenter survey. Birth Berkeley Calif. March 2021;48(1):61 -5.

84. Guise JM, Eden K, Emeis C, Denman MA, Marshall N, Fu RR, et al. Vaginal birth after cesarean: new insights. Evid ReportTechnology Assess. March 2010;(191):1-

397.

85. Leung AS, Leung EK, Paul RH. Uterine rupture after previous cesarean delivery: maternal and fetal consequences. Am J Obstet Gynecol. Oct 1993;169(4):945-50.

86. Royal College of Obstetricians and Gynecologists. Birth after previous Caesarian birth. Green-Top Guideline, 2007 (www.rcog.org.uk).

87. Guiliano M, Closset E, Therby D, LeGoueff F, Deruelle P, Subtil D. Signs, symptoms and complications of complete and partial uterine ruptures during pregnancy and delivery. Eur J Obstet Gynecol Reprod Biol. aout 2014; 179:130-4.

88. Arulkumaran S, Chua S, Ratnam SS. Symptoms and signs with scar rupture--value of uterine activity measurements. Obstet Gynaecol. August 1992;32(3):208-12.

89. Cunningham FG. Cunningham FG, MacDonald PC, Gout NF, Leveno KJ, Gilstrap LC. Injuries to the birth canal. In: Williams Obstetrics. 19th Ed. Prentice-Hall International Inc; 1993, p. 543-53.

90. Amate P, Aflak N, Luton D. Uterine rupture during pregnancy. EMC Obstet 2014 ;10 [5-080-A-10].

91. perrotin F, Marret H, Lansac J. Uterus cicatriciel : la revision systématique de la cicatrice de cesarienne apres accouchement par voie vaginale est-elle toujours utile?J Gynecol Obstet Biol Reprod 1999; 28:253-62.

92. Wang YL, Su TH. Obstetric uterine rupture of the unscarred uterus: a twenty-year clinical analysis. Gynecol Obstet Invest. 2006 ;62(3) :131-5.

93. Kaabar H. Kaabar H. Uterine rupture during labour. These Medecine Tunis 1990:86.

94. Barger MK, Weiss J, Nannini A, Werler M, Heeren T, Stubblefield PG. Risk factors for uterine rupture among women who attempt a vaginal birth after a previous cesarean: a case-control study. J Reprod Med. August 2011;56(7-8):313-20.

95. Delarue T,Pele P. Prevention des ruptures et pre ruptures des uterus anterieurement cesarises, a propos de 14 observations. J Gynecol Obstet biol reprod 1981;10;3:259-67.

96. Guyot A, Carbonnel M, Frey C, Pharisien I, Uzan M, Carbillon L. Uterine rupture: risk factors, maternal and fetal complications. J Gynecologie Obstetrique Biol Reprod. May 2010;39(3):238-45.

97. Koulimaya-Gombet CE, Diouf AA, Diallo M, Dia A, Sene C, Moreau JC, et al. Pregnancy and delivery in patients with antecedent cesarean section in Dakar: epidemio-clinical therapeutical and prognostic aspects. Pan Afr Med J. 22 June 2017; 27:135.

98. Thakur A, Heer MS, Thakur V, Heer GK, Narone JN, Narone RK. Subtotal hysterectomy for uterine rupture. Int J Gynaecol Obstet Off Organ Int Fed Gynaecol Obstet. July 2001;74(1):29-33.

99. Ofir K, Sheiner E, Levy A, Katz M, Mazor M. Uterine rupture: differences between a scarred and an unscarred uterus. Am J Obstet Gynecol. Aout2004;191(2):425-9.

100. Njim S. Les ruptures uterines a la maternite du CHU de Monastir a propos de 32 cas. These Med Sfax 1990.

101. Nkwey L,Tozin R,Umba T. evolution of ruptures of the gravid uterus in the university clinics of kinshasa .J Gynecol Obstet Biol Reprod 1983;12;7:755- 61.

102. Voogd LB, Wood HB, Powell DV. Ruptured uterus. Obstet Gynecol. Jan 1956;7(1):70-7.

103. Diemunsch P, Pottecher J, Chassard D. Elements de la prise en charge anesthesique en cas d'antecedent de cesarienne. J Gynecologie Obstetrique Biol Reprod. Dec 2012;41(8):817-21.

104. GoffinetF, MercierF, TeyssierV, PierreF, DreyfusM, MignonA, et al.Hemorrhages du post-partum: recommandations du CNGOF pour la pratique clinique (decembre2004). Gynecol Obstet Fertil 2005;33:268-74.

105. Bollaert, P. R., Annane, D'Aube, H., Bedos, J. P., Cariou, A., Du Cheyron, D Lutun, P. (2002). Disseminated intravascular coagulation (DIC) in intensive care: definition, classification and treatment (with the exception of cancer and malignant hemopathies). Reanimation, 11(8), 567-574.

106. Schrinsky DC, Benson RC. Rupture of the pregnant uterus: a review. Obstet Gynecol Surv. Apr 1978;33(4):217-32.

107. Drira M. La rupture uterine a l'hopital universitaire Habib Thameur de Tunis, 1960a 1982.These de medecine; Tunis1983;n1231.

108. Zelop CM, Harlow BL, Frigoletto FD, Safon LE, Saltzman DH. Emergency peripartum hysterectomy. Am J Obstet Gynecol. May 1993;168(5):1443-8.

109. Yap OW, Kim ES, Laros RK. Maternal and neonatal outcomes after uterine rupture in labor. Am J Obstet Gynecol. June 2001;184(7):1576-81.

110. Chamiso B. Rupture of pregnant uterus in Shashemene General Hospital, south Shoa, Ethiopia (a three year study of 57 cases). Ethiop Med J. Oct 1995;33(4):251-7.

111. Soltan MH, Khashoggi T, Adelusi B. Pregnancy following rupture of the pregnant uterus. Int J Gynecol Obstet. Jan 1996;52(1):37-42.

112. Boutaleb y., Aderdour m., Zhiri ma. Boutaleb y., Aderdour m., Zhiri ma. Les ruptures uterines J. Gynecol. Obstet. Biol. Repr, 1982,11:87-89.

113. Champaul G. Ruptures uterines. African experience of 64 cases J.Gynecol.Ostet. Biol.- Reprod1978, 7,4855-860.

114. Drabo A. Les ruptures uterines a l'hopital Somine Dolo de Mopti: facteurs influengant le pronostic materno foetal et mesures prophylactiques a propos de 25 cas. These de Medecine Bamako .2000, N°7.

115. Ozdemir I, Yucel N, Yucel O. Rupture of the pregnant uterus: a 9-year review. Arch Gynecol Obstet. Sept 2005;272(3):229-31.

116. Diallo f.b. Vangeenderhuysen, D. baraka, i. Hadiza, Sahabi, i. labo, m. dare, m. garba.la rupture uterine a la maternite centrale de reference de Niamey (Niger) Aspects epidemiologiques et stratégies de prévention. Medecine d'Afrique Noire: 1998, 45 (5).

117. Attalah K. A propos de 37 cas de ruptures uterines observes a la maternite de l'hopital Charles Nicolle du 01/01/74 au 31/12/79. These Medecine Tunis 1984; n 35.

118. Cahill AG, Stamilio DM, Odibo AO, Peipert JF, Ratcliffe SJ, Stevens EJ, et al. Is vaginal birth after cesarean (VBAC) or elective repeat cesarean safer in women with a prior vaginal delivery? Am J Obstet Gynecol. Oct 2006;195(4):1143-7.

119. Abauleth (y R. ), ABAULETH (Y.R.), KOFFI (A.K.), CISSE (M.L.), BONI (S.). Prognosis of uterine rupture during labour: A propos de 293 cas colliges au chu de Bouake (Cote D'ivoire). Med Trop (Mars) [Internet]. 2006 [cite 9 sept 2022]

120. Sepou A, Yanza MC, Nguembi E, Ngbale R, Kouriah G, Kouabosso A, et al. Uterine rupture in the maternity ward of the Bangui Community Hospital (Central

Africa). Med Trop Rev Corps Sante Colon. 2002;62(5):517-20.

121.    INSERM, sante publique France / Maternal deaths in France: better understanding for better prevention. 6th report of the National Confidential Enquiry into Maternal Deaths (ENCMM) 2013-2015.

122.    Kieser KE, Baskett TF. A 10-year population-based study of uterine rupture. Obstet Gynecol. Oct 2002;100(4):749-53.

123.    Taleb Zadeh H. Les ruptures uterines a l'hopital shahpour de Tabriz. Rev Fr Gynecol Obstet 1978;73:695-702.

124.    Tinsa F., Gherissi A. Tinsa F., Gherissi A Les services de sante de la reproduction: satisfaction ou insatisfaction? Unite de Recherche Evaluation en Sante. Faculte de Medecine de Tunis. 2012.

125.    Recommandation pratique clinique: accouchement sur uterus cicatriciel.36es journees nationales Paris, 2012 [Internet]. 12 Sep 2022. Available at: http://www.cngof.fr/pratiques-cliniques/recommandations-pour-la-pratique-clinique?folder=RPC%2BCOLLEGE%252F2012

126.    Diaz SD, Jones JE, Seryakov M, Mann WJ. Uterine rupture and dehiscence: ten- year review and case-control study. South Med J. Apr2002; 95(4):431 -5.

127.    Sayed Ahmed WA, Habash YH, Hamdy MA, Ghoneim HM. Rupture of the pregnant uterus - a 20-year review. J Matern Fetal Neonatal Med. 18 June 2017;30(12):1488-93.

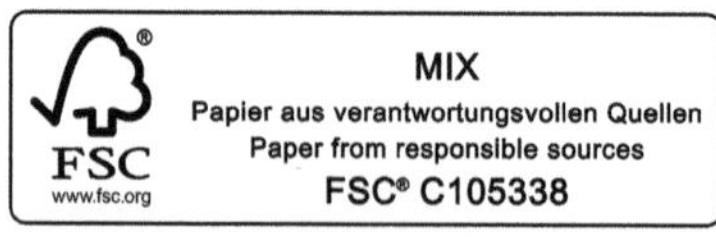

Printed by Books on Demand GmbH, Norderstedt / Germany